Shape up with

GABBY
ALLEN

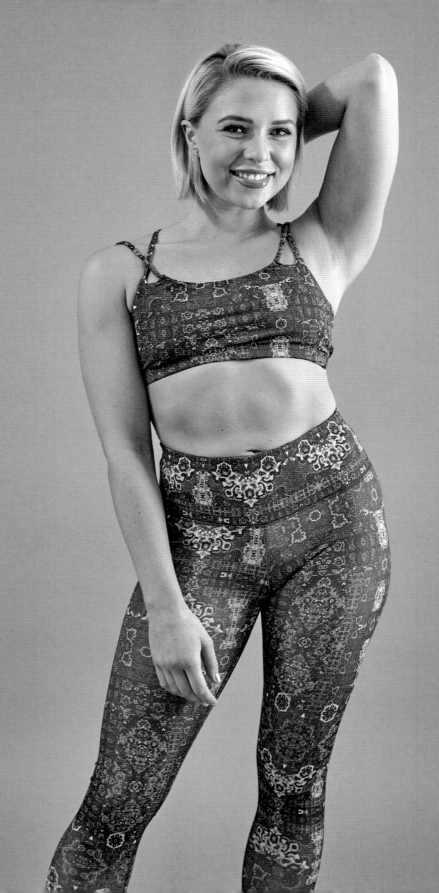

Shape up with
GABBY ALLEN

Fast food and dynamic workouts

—

Transform your body in **4 weeks**

EBURY
PRESS

Acknowledgements

I never imagined I would be lucky enough to write a book – it was always a goal up there and now it's a dream come true thanks to an incredible team.

I will be forever grateful for my team at United Agents. The book wouldn't exist if it wasn't for them believing I could do it and doing everything in their power to make sure I did do it! Ariella, your words of wisdom and advice, Matt and Harry, your support and encouragement, gave me the confidence to do this.

The lovely Kate Faithful-Williams, you are a dream! Thank you for spending hours upon hours listening to me, most definitely, delve into stories that were 100% were not appropriate for the book. You listened with interest and enthusiasm, and I proudly now call you a friend. Your input and creativity has given the book that extra flare and I am very lucky to have worked with you on it.

Laura at Ebury, thank you for your patience and 'hands-on' work throughout! I loved having you at the shoot, talking AND walking through the workouts with me. You really have been a highlight in the whole process for me. Thank you to Steph, Chloe, Helen and the rest of the wonderful team at Ebury. I feel blessed to have worked with such a hard working but thoroughly kind group of people.

Thank you to Mike English for your beautiful photography. Your passion for your work is so apparent and made it a joy to work with you. And to Louise Evans for designing my book. It is everything I wanted and more.

Thank you to my friends for your grounding and humbling nature. I am very lucky to have such loyal, inspiring people in my life.

Finally, I would like to thank my mum and brother. It's down to their on-going strength and determination that I am where I am today. I appreciate you both so much, you inspire me every day to be the best version of myself and my main goal in life is to do you proud. You've put up with my hopes and dreams since forever. Thanks to you, and Dad, I am gradually climbing towards them. I am so grateful, Mum, for all you have done for me, for giving me the discipline to go to dance classes, for cheering me on during fitness ventures. You have always been my biggest fan, and believe it or not, I am yours!

To everybody involved, you're wonderful. None of it would be possible without all of you. Thank you.

1 3 5 7 9 10 8 6 4 2

Published in 2019 by Ebury Press an imprint of Ebury Publishing, 20 Vauxhall Bridge Road, London SW1V 2SA

Ebury Press is part of the Penguin Random House group of companies whose addresses can be found at global.penguinrandomhouse.com

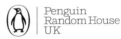

Penguin Random House UK

First published by Ebury Press in 2019

www.penguin.co.uk

A CIP catalogue record for this book is available from the British Library

ISBN 978 1 529 10416 5

Colour origination by Altaimage, London
Printed and bound in Italy by L.E.G.O. S.p.A

Penguin Random House is committed to a sustainable future for our business, our readers and our planet.

This book is made from Forest Stewardship Council® certified paper.

MIX
Paper from responsible sources
FSC® C018179

Contents

Hello

Thank you for picking up this book!

So, I'm going to be honest with you right from the start: I work hard to stay in shape. I'm not naturally really slim; it would be a joke if I pretended that I was. I'm the short girl who used to envy slim friends with legs that go on and on; friends who have flat tummies despite eating three cakes a day. Like, HOW?! How is that even possible? I'm guessing you've opened up this book because you're like me – and you want to look and feel your best too.

The framework for this book came together in Mallorca, just down the road from the *Love Island* villa. It was such an exciting time because I was about to go on the show, but also nerve-wracking and... kinda boring. Being in lockdown for two weeks, babysat by my chaperone, meant I had literally nothing to do.

So I made my own fun. I didn't have weights with me and there was no chance of going out to a class, so I invented my own high-energy bodyweight workouts. I'm not exaggerating at all when I say these workouts saved my sanity and made me feel completely confident striding into the *Love Island* villa.

It was surreal when a 'bombshell' islander coming into the villa dropped a hint from the outside world: people were talking about my abs. 'There's even a hashtag #gabsabs.' I was like, what? Amazing! That's the kind of results I want you to get too.

I promise I can help you burn fat and tone and sculpt your body so you feel like the very best version of yourself. I fully expect that, if you stick to the plan, in four weeks time you'll have toned up your legs, you'll have more visible abs and you'll drop a dress size. You'll feel more confident in your clothes – and out of your clothes. It won't be easy, but it will be worth it.

If you already have my app or have worked out with one of my online classes, the moves here will be familiar but the weekly plan and exercise combinations will be new to you – you gotta vary your workouts to keep them interesting. Once you're familiar with all the moves, mix up your workouts yourself to stay motivated.

What I've also got you here, which I'm really excited to share, are 60 recipes and an eating plan to combine with your workouts to maximise your results.

Eating is one of the things I get asked most often about by my clients – what should I eat to get in shape? What's healthy? So here is my guide to eating to feel fit without dieting and losing your social life!!

I'm a personal trainer, not a chef, so the recipes here are really simple. They are based on what I eat and the eating principles that work for me – lots of lean protein, lots of veg, low on carbohydrates, not too much sugar and only from natural sources like fruit and honey. I love a cheese burger, I love ice cream, I get takeaways... I'm human OK? But when I want to look and feel my best, the food here is what I turn to.

With these healthy and simple recipes, you can work towards the body you want without going hungry. I learned the hard way that complicated diets are not sustainable, so in this book there's no calorie-counting (the recipes are naturally lower in calories). No miserable weigh-ins that make you feel like crap. And you can still go out and have a laugh.

This book is all about eating to feel good while still living your life.

What I really love about being a personal trainer is that I can help you build your confidence as much as I can help you get in better shape. With this book, I'm here to motivate and guide you every step of the way – what to eat and how to work out but also how to party and peel yourself up off the couch when you've lost your motivation too. It happens to the best of us; sometimes I can't be arsed either.

I hope you love the recipes and workouts as much as I do. And I know you'll love your results even more.

Gabby
xx

My promise to you

Shape Up is all about how good it makes you feel. That's no wishy-washy promise. In four weeks you're going to feel:

- **Physically transformed:** you could drop a dress size, tone your legs and discover your abs hiding inside;

- **Stronger:** mentally and physically, you'll have the kick-ass strength to reach your goals;

- **Motivated:** all my workouts and recipes are designed to give you energy so you want to come back for more;

- **Empowered:** you'll understand the foods and fitness routine that your body needs, and you have the tools right here to make it happen;

- **Confident in your skin:** in these pages, I believe you'll discover the best version of yourself.

What does being 'in shape' really mean?

One word: *Confidence!*

How this book works

Over the next month, I'll coach you through five workouts a week. If that sounds like waaaay more exercise than you're used to, don't worry. I'm here to cheer you on.

I've used all my years of dance and personal training to make every workout fire up your endorphin high, sculpt your body from every angle and get you hooked on that exercise afterglow.

I don't have much time to cook so the recipes here are quick, faff-free and yum. Every day, you're going to enjoy three energising, protein-packed, home-cooked meals.

Plus, I want you to structure in my smart snack options. Weirdly, I've found the secret to eating well is to never go hungry. But you do need to be prepared so you don't reach for a bag of crisps or sugary snack bar when you're hungry, so I've shared my top tips for meal-prepping and snack-packing.

I think you'll start seeing results in the first fortnight. If you have a wobble – and because you're normal, you will – ask yourself this: why did you pick up this book?

Always remember how good you feel after a workout, and how happy you feel after eating an amazing, healthy meal that you threw together yourself.

Whether you're on this four-week plan to feel like your old self again, to look your best in a bikini or even to make your ex regret the day they messed you around, I believe this book will shape up your body and your whole life.

Why are you reading my book? – Because you want to shape up, and I believe you can do it.

My s.h.a.p.e. philosophy

Sweat your feelings out

Challenge yourself with your exercise routine,
and you'll get results before you've even completed
the four weeks.

Hit your happy shape

Forget scales and calorie-counting: focus on shaping
up your mind as much as your body, so you feel more
confident being exactly who you are.

Activate endorphins

Yeah, it's satisfying to look hot, but the best thing
about shaping up is how it makes you feel. Work out
for the natural chemical high, not just to burn fat,
and you'll keep motivated and enjoy the process
a whole lot more.

Party on

I love going out. You can stay healthy even when you
fancy a drink and there's no way you want to miss
dinner with your friends.

Enjoy food

Choose wisely so you're eating what makes your body
feel good. Make sure what you're eating is full of flavour
and easy to prep.

Why I love to sweat my feelings out

Fitness is therapy for me. When I'm stressed about something or my boyfriend's winding me up, exercise gets all that negativity out! Throwing punches with a boxing circuit or busting out a round of burpees releases the frustration.

When you're obsessing over a problem and it spins round and round your head, exercise helps you escape that head fuck. Because it's hard to think about anything else when you're working so hard, you're sweating your heart out.

Working out is a kind of mindfulness: you're completely in the moment. And by the end of the workout, when you're drenched in sweat, you realise you've not thought about that stupid row you had with your mate, that never-ending work project or that Instagram post that got zero likes. It gives you a huge lift and a bit of perspective.

Exercise always makes me feel good about myself. Before I went into *Love Island* I was so nervous, I didn't know what to expect at all. I worried I was making a big mistake. So while the producers of the show had me in lockdown in Majorca – two weeks without my phone, I repeat WITHOUT MY PHONE 😱 or speaking to anyone except my chaperone – I did my own workouts and my mood lifted higher and higher every day. By the time I walked onto the set for the first time, I felt amazing.

When life gets rocky, fitness is the therapy that pulls me through. When boyfriends have cheated on me, I'm tempted to do a Bridget Jones and eat my body weight in ice cream. Instead, when I break up with someone, I consciously think: 'Fuck you, I'm going to make myself even better than when you were with me.' So I hit the gym with a vengeance. Working out is the best way for me to get over a non-deserving ex and get myself feeling amazing. And posting that first bikini picture is always a winner. Ha!

Fitness is such fantastic therapy for me that I became a personal trainer as a way of taking control of my life. Until I educated myself about taking care of my body, I was chasing my tail juggling four jobs, frustrated with living in a grotty flat and stuck in a relationship that was going nowhere. My passion for fitness led to *Love Island*, to creating my own business and a whole life that I love. Read this book, make yourself feel better physically, inject yourself with some fresh energy and renew your zest for life.

How I finally hit my happy shape

My weight went up and down like a yo-yo before I hit my happy shape. It took a long time, so this section is the longest read. Well, 5 minutes. But maybe reading this will save you the years I spent obsessively dieting, and help you get your happy shape.

As a teenager, I got the idea that I had to look a certain way: skinny. I believed that being any bigger than a size 8 would be a disaster. I was at drama school in London, and my dream was to be a dancer. I'd been dancing since I was three years old and being on stage was all I ever wanted. My drama school teachers never actually came out and said, 'You need to be thin if you want to make it.' But teachers would comment on your weight. If a girl in the class lost a few pounds, they'd say, 'You're looking really good at the moment, have you lost weight?' I had it in my head that being skinny = looking good. I was permanently on a diet. But the diets were so extreme they were impossible to stick to.

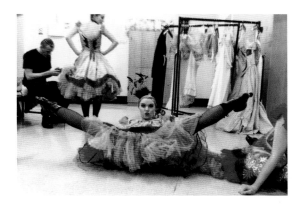

Living the dream at drama school!

Then suddenly, I lost a lot of weight. And it had nothing to do with dieting. My dad was very sick with brain cancer. He was my rock, and over a year he got weaker and weaker. Every time I got the train back to our family home in Ecclestone, just outside Liverpool, Dad seemed to have shrunk a little smaller.

When he died, me, my mum and brother Ethan were knocked sideways by grief. I couldn't eat, couldn't sleep, couldn't find the joy in anything. I felt completely lost. So it was weird when I went back to drama school and people said, 'Wow, you've lost weight, you look great.' In fact, it was plain wrong. I felt absolutely miserable.

But I was mixed up. I was grieving over my dad, and unable to think straight. It took me years to figure out the pattern: when I'm at my thinnest, I am unhappy.

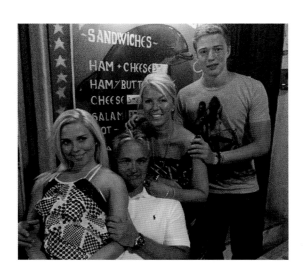

Dad, me, mum and Ethan x

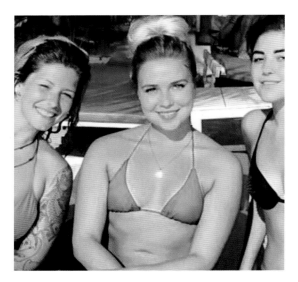

Yo-yo dieting days...

My weight continued to yo-yo up and down for the next few years. I compared myself to friends and other dancers. Auditioning against girls who were slimmer than me knocked my confidence. I often felt uncomfortable in my clothes and I'd be like, 'Right, I need to sort this out now.' Looking back I can see that I didn't get those gigs or that guy because I didn't believe in myself; it wasn't because of my weight.

I took dieting too far because I was so hung up on what the scales said. I remember one Christmas, right after a really painful breakup, I was training too much and not eating anywhere near enough. I had no body fat. My boobs had gone. I came back home and my mum and brother looked at me in utter horror. They said I'd lost too much weight and didn't look well.

It was only when the people I care about most in the world told me I looked ill that I realised I needed to start taking care of myself. That's when I decided to qualify as a personal trainer: to learn how to look after my own body first and then help other people give their bodies a whole lot of love too.

When I started getting really into exercise, the first thing people noticed was that I had a glow about me. An energy. A sense that I'm happy in my body. That's the best feeling. I'm proud of having an active, fit body: all the training I put in shows. Having abs and a sculpted butt takes effort, but it's fun and it makes you feel confident inside.

The best thing anyone can ever say to me is, 'You look healthy.' Not, 'You look skinny.' Healthy is the best look. It comes with a glow, a bounce, because happiness is far more than your physical shape: it's a feeling inside.

The most body confident I've ever been was right before I went into *Love Island*. I was in the absolute prime of training. I had abs for days! I was training five days a week and I felt fab in and out of my clothes.

So what I'm saying is this: shaping up isn't all about weight loss. In this book, I want to help you hit your happy shape by giving your body the exercise and food you need to feel your best. It's all here.

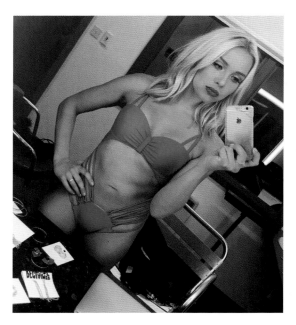

When my abs had a hashtag!

How to activate endorphins

**Maybe you see working out as a necessary evil. Something you *have*
to do, not something you *want* to do. So let me tell you a little secret:
sometimes I dread exercise too.**

'How do you stay motivated?' is one
of the questions I get asked every day on
Instagram. Every. Single. Day. We all
struggle with it. So what I do is this:

1. Dream up a load of stupid excuses
    about why I can't exercise;

2. Remember how good I feel after
    a workout;

3. Tell those excuses to do one and start
    warming up.

Sometimes before a workout, I'm not joking,
I literally want to kill every single person I
know, then after my session I finish feeling
like, 'Hugs! Rainbows! Puppies! Unicorns!
I love you!' Because the endorphin high you
get after a workout is insane. Moving your
body is the best feeling.

When I'm feeling lazy, in the back of my
mind I've got my small 12-year-old self, who
went from being a prize-winning ballerina to
being bedbound. I had severe scoliosis, a
condition where my spine had grown so
wonky that I had to have two steel rods
surgically implanted to straighten me out.

I woke up in intensive care after the
operation and felt like I'd been snapped
in half, like a plank of wood. The pain
was intense.

Two weeks later, I started walking again
and, though I was wobbly and in pain, the
more I moved, the better I felt. After a few
months I was back at dance class, and
within a year I won the North West ballet
championship. The next year I went to the
all-England ballet finals.

I think having that setback made me work
harder. My scar is 40cm long, from the base
of my skull all the way down to my bottom.
It's a permanent reminder to appreciate the
simple joy of moving my body.

Being physically strong makes me feel
more confident. With every workout I not
only build my physical strength, but I feel
more positive. Sometimes I have to really
dig deep to push through a round of press-
ups, but afterwards I feel superhuman. Like,
there's *nothing* I can't do. Exercise activates
a natural endorphin high, and it's yours for
the taking.

With every workout I feel more positive

Why I party on

I love going out. I genuinely think it's healthy to cut loose.

I've been on many a diet that's come unstuck by trying to be too 'clean'. I've been through phases of trying to live on nothing but vegetables and early nights. I've cut out everything from carbs to solid food. I've starved myself on juice fasts, trying to eat as little as humanly possible. It's so boring. Result: I rebel. All the wine! More wine! Let's go clubbing! Chips and gravy on the way home!

So the day after a 'clean' trip to the farmers' market, I'd be severely hungover and go to the greasy spoon. I'd eat everything that you could possibly fry and fit on a plate. And give me the biggest plate you've got, please. And three rounds of toast. Can you imagine going to the gym after that? No way.

Life doesn't have to be all or nothing. There are sacrifices I'm not prepared to make for amazing abs. Going out, for one. My lifestyle has to accommodate that, because my friends and family are so important to me.

I like having a good time – I don't want to always be the one who's like, 'No, I can't eat that,' and 'No, I'm not drinking.' And I love lying around on the sofa watching TV of an evening; I can't be arsed to meditate, mess around with pond-scum smoothies or go to bed at 9pm. My life is more important to me. It's cringe to say it, but YOLO.

After a night out, I now wake up in the morning ready to work out, not ready to die. On page 24 I've got you a whole section on what I order when I'm out for dinner, exactly what I drink and how much (Sorry, Mum). And if you do overdo it, flip to page 45 for my favourite healthy hangover breakfast recipe.

Life doesn't have to be all or nothing

My journey to enjoying food

I haven't always had a healthy relationship with food. I binged. I'd stick rigidly to some ridiculous diet for maybe three weeks, then find myself in the corner shop loading up on spicy crisps, family-sized packets of chocolate digestives and giant bags of sweets because I was so hungry. Junk food was the ultimate quick fix for that stupid quick-fix-fad diet. Or I'd get a Chinese takeaway and order the whole of China.

The weight always came back on.

But the real trouble with fad diets is that you don't actually think about what you're eating, so pretty quickly your body is going to go, 'Aaaaaargh, WTF?' and make you eat EVERYTHING. If you want to stay in shape you have to make it easy for your body and mind to live healthily for a lifetime.

That means forgiving yourself for little hiccups along the way. It doesn't mean getting into a whole spiral of 'treats' and 'cheating'.

I know that when I have sugar in my house, it gets eaten. By me. Biscuits burn a hole in my cupboard.

You need quick, easy recipes you can put in your belly in less than 10 minutes so you don't crave biscuits! You need enough natural sweetness so you never feel deprived, and the right balance of protein, healthy fats and good carbs so you'll feel satisfied. I've paid attention to portion control in all the recipes so you won't feel hungry or uncomfortably full.

Now I've made my healthy eating easy, I don't descend into binge mode. I know I can knock up a healthy meal in a hurry, so I don't grab at junk in the shop. I enjoy my food and I'm happy with my body. You can get there too.

Tracking your progress

I'm not a fan of weigh-ins, and I don't have scales in my house. There are healthier ways to track your progress and I'd like you to try, because when you look back in four weeks time I know you're going to be impressed with what you've achieved.

Here's how to track your shape up story:

1. On the day you start this plan, take two selfies: front on and sideways;

2. Take a photo on the same day every week, first thing in the morning.

3. If you're sticking to your training plan and eating three meals a day from my menu of healthy fast food, by week four, you'll see the difference.

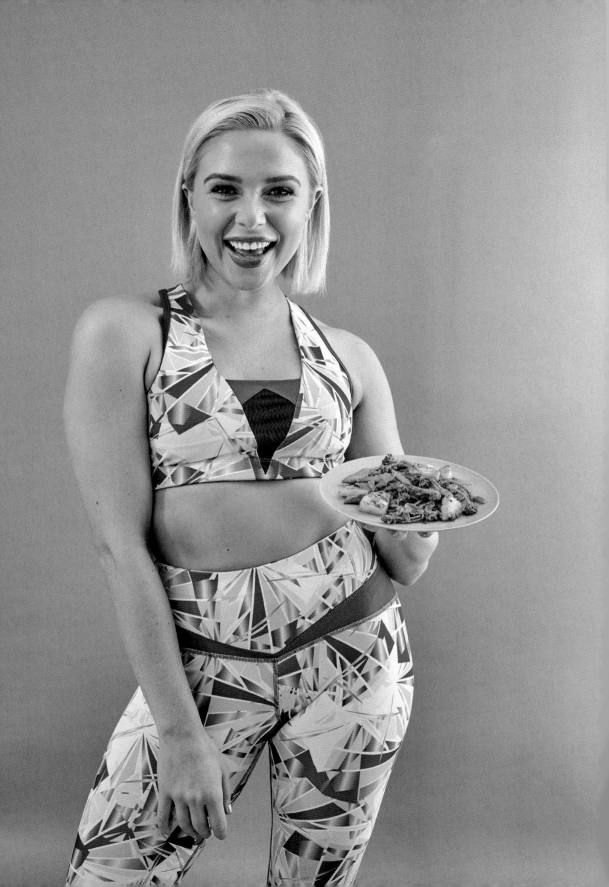

Hungry?

Let's talk about food...

Life can be pretty crazy, so taking the hassle out of healthy eating makes shaping up a whole lot easier.

I'm a hungry person. If you train as much as I do – and you will! – then you need to eat well.

You'll find no faffy methods, no weird ingredients and no complicated instructions here, just fresh, satisfying food that tastes good.

Your essential menu, on a plate:

LOTS OF...

Lean protein, like chicken, steak, prawns, cod and turkey bacon

Colourful vegetables in every shade of the rainbow

JUST ENOUGH...

Natural sweeteners, like honey

Healthy fats, including avocado and egg yolks, which help your body absorb vitamins

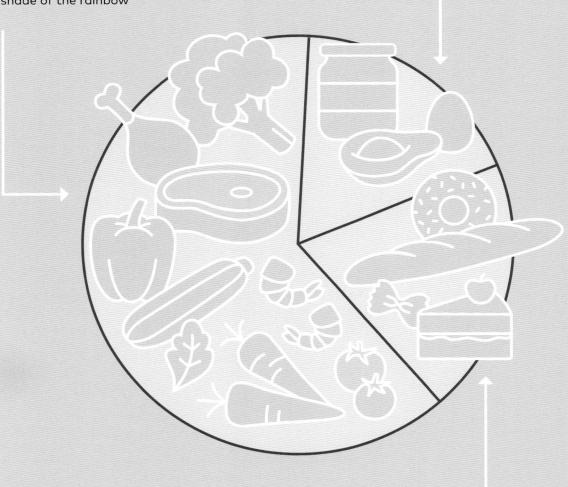

Keep it simple: your menu doesn't discriminate between workout days and rest days because it's important to eat lean protein and colourful vegetables every day. Don't complicate things.

CUTTING DOWN ON...

Processed carbs, like bread, pasta and cake

My 7 top tips:

1. Map your meals

What are you going to eat, and what time? Don't leave it to chance: you're going to be hungry every three or four hours so map out breakfast, lunch, snack (see more on snack control on page 119) and dinner every day.

If you get too hungry, you'll only end up eating crap. I've been there. If I don't plan ahead and get hungry, I choose badly and I quickly notice my waistline expanding. Weirdly, I don't get in shape by eating less, but by eating better food.

2. Shop supermarket superfoods

It really annoys me when healthy food is ridiculously expensive. It doesn't have to be that way. But if you want to eat better food, then you do need to cook from scratch.

In my recipes, I celebrate supermarket superfoods, like blueberries, peanut butter, cashews and Greek yogurt, chicken, fish, steak, eggs, chillies, broccoli, kale, tomatoes, mushrooms. When you fill your kitchen with these healthy ingredients, it's easy to throw a nutritious meal together in minutes.

3. Ditch cheats

I don't want cheats in my life, whether they're bad boyfriends or cheat days. At first, the idea of a whole day where you can eat EVERYTHING sounds great. But the reality is, cheat days make getting in shape harder because you'll crave the 'treats' you eat on your 'cheat' days on other days and you'll get stuck in a cycle of over-eating on one day and depriving yourself for the rest

– better to break the habits and eat better every day. In *Big Brother* we didn't have sugar for a week. When we got biscuits back in the house again, I'd lost the taste for biscuits and sugar. Sweet victory!

I understand you might really want chocolate one day. That's OK. Just one piece of advice: enjoy that chocolate. Don't punish yourself for it. You're not counting down the days of deprivation until you can blow out and eat the whole world. Instead, you are eating well every day and educating yourself about how to negotiate daily temptations – more on those later.

4. Drink up

Aim to drink at least 3 litres of water a day. Avoid juices and fizzy drinks because they're basically liquid sugar. I love a Diet Coke, but if you're shaping up, water is what your body needs. And water gives you more energy than any so-called 'sports drink' will.

Fill up a bottle and start the habit now: if you always have water with you, you'll sip it continually. Result: glowy skin, more energy, you're flushing out toxins and, water can help break the 'I'm bored, I need a snack' habit.

When I feel that urge to prowl around for a snack, my mum taught me to drink water first. Most of the time when you think you're hungry, you're not: you're actually thirsty. Does that make you reach for a drink of water now? Yeah it does! Then, if you're still hungry in half an hour, you know it's time to eat.

If you still want a little something between meals to keep you going, add a snack or dessert (pages 118–135) – don't hold back and feel hungry. You can prep them in advance and stash them in your bag.

5. Portion caution

I don't recommend counting calories or grams of fat as it can make you kinda obsessive. Trust me, I know from experience! But it really is worth paying attention to portion size. Because even if you're eating whole foods like avocado, if you're putting away a mountain of them then you're consuming way more than you need. A quarter of avocado with lunch is great; half an avocado over the day is plenty. An avocado a day is too much of a good thing.

A GUIDE TO PORTION SIZES...

• **Meat:** palm of your hand;

• **Fish:** your outstretched hand;

• **Fat:** palm of your hand;

• **Healthy carbs:** palm of your hand;

• **Non-starchy veg (avoid beige veg and eat the rainbow instead):** as much as you like.

ARE YOU VEGAN?

I'm not vegan myself, but if you don't eat meat, fish, eggs or dairy I've suggested vegan versions of over half of my recipes. I'm going to trust that you've done all the research on getting enough protein in your diet though.

6. Healthy carbs & healthy fat

Carbs are not the devil. But cutting down on processed carbs, like bread, cereal and cake, will give you more energy, not to mention visible abs. I focus on healthy carbs: vegetables, pulses and wholegrains.

I'm usually not a fan of low-fat versions of yogurt, cream cheese or whatever, because when manufacturers remove the fat they often add sugar to make the product taste good. Also, when the fat is reduced, you may find you're left wanting more. So, I eat the glorious, filling, full-fat versions of yogurt, cream cheese, hummus, peanut butter, Cheddar, the works. Try it.

A special note on Greek yogurt: traditional Greek yogurt has the protein we're looking for: 9g per 100g. Choose this over 'Greek-style', flavoured or low-fat Greek yogurt.

7. Shop & chop Sunday

If you've got healthy food in the fridge ready to go, you've got a healthy body ready to go too. I'm a big believer in meal prep and batch cooking, so on Sundays I'll do a big shop and chop of my healthy ingredients. I roast veggies for lunchboxes and quick dinners, prep breakfasts when I need to dash out the door and make my snacks in advance too. When you're all set up for a healthy week, it's so much easier to stick to the plan.

Let's talk overeating

Knowing when to stop is a massive thing for all of us. We're conditioned by our nans to finish our plates, even if we feel uncomfortably full. I hate that 'Omigod I can't move' feeling, lying horizontal on the sofa with my jeans undone. In the past I've cancelled nights out because I feel so full and tired after dinner.

Ways to help avoid feeling this full:

Pause: Enjoy chatting to your mates while you're eating. You may find that putting your knife and fork down during conversation gives your brain a chance to realise that your tummy's full.

Stop: Pay attention to how strong you feel when you know you've had your fill. Willpower is a muscle, and the more you exercise it, the stronger it gets.

Fast forward: You know how you motivate yourself to exercise by remembering the post-workout afterglow? Flip it. I've had enough biscuit binges to know I always feel terrible afterwards. Maybe you've been there too. Save yourself that regret and distract yourself with something better: Netflix? Exercise? Sex? You choose.

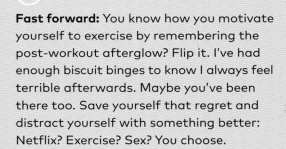

I've had enough biscuit binges to know I always feel terrible afterwards

Is it possible to party & stay in shape?

One word: yes. You need highlights in your life. Hanging out with friends is a healthy habit – you have a laugh, you're with people who totally get you, you're not eating alone in front of the TV. So here's what to do:

When you're out for dinner... I like to look at the menu in advance so I can make a smart decision about what to order before I get there and not get swayed into something that's not so healthy. I'll choose something that's high in protein, with healthy carbs and lots of fresh goodness. Try to choose something that resembles one of the recipes in this book, like steak with tenderstem broccoli and sweet potato chunky chips, or cod on a bed of baby carrots and buttered greens.

When you fancy dessert... Have dessert. I've found it's healthier having dessert when you're out instead of at home because you can share it with a friend. Most importantly, when you're eating out you won't find yourself accidentally wandering into the restaurant kitchen to polish off another portion. At home that could easily happen!

When you're up for a drink... I like to go out, so to stay in shape I take the most sugary booze – beer, wine, dark spirits – off the menu. I order a vodka soda with fresh lime (not cordial). Occasionally I'll have a prosecco, but I find I know where I'm at with vodka:

- The soda water is hydrating, which takes the edge right off a hangover;

- You taste the spirit, so you're more aware of how much you're drinking;

- You can order a single shot and finish it – your glass isn't topped up without you realising;

- The clearer the drink, the fewer sugary calories.

How many vodkas are ok? Enough until you're on the floor. Jokes. Realistically, I have about six units on a night out. Yes, Mum, that's more than the NHS recommends. Guilty. I apply the rule: remember how you feel afterwards. Would morning-after me regret a seventh drink? Bleurrrgh. I would. I know when to stop on a night out so I can get going with a workout tomorrow.

If you want to shape up, you have to pick and choose.

How to re-set if you fall off the wagon

Climb back on the wagon today with an extra workout. Use my recipes to plan your meals for the week ahead and get a load of healthy shopping in.

It will feel good to get back to eating well. I fell off the healthy wagon in the *Big Brother* house, with little to do but eat biscuits and potatoes for a whole month. I felt like a potato: round, pale and spotty. I swear I had a maximum of four vegetables the whole time I was in there. My skin was awful, I felt tired all the time, and every week I felt more out of shape. 'Frustrated' doesn't begin to describe it.

When I got back into the real world, I was like, 'Please, give me broccoli! I need nutrients!' If you fall off the wagon, re-setting is the best feeling.

Re-setting is the best feeling

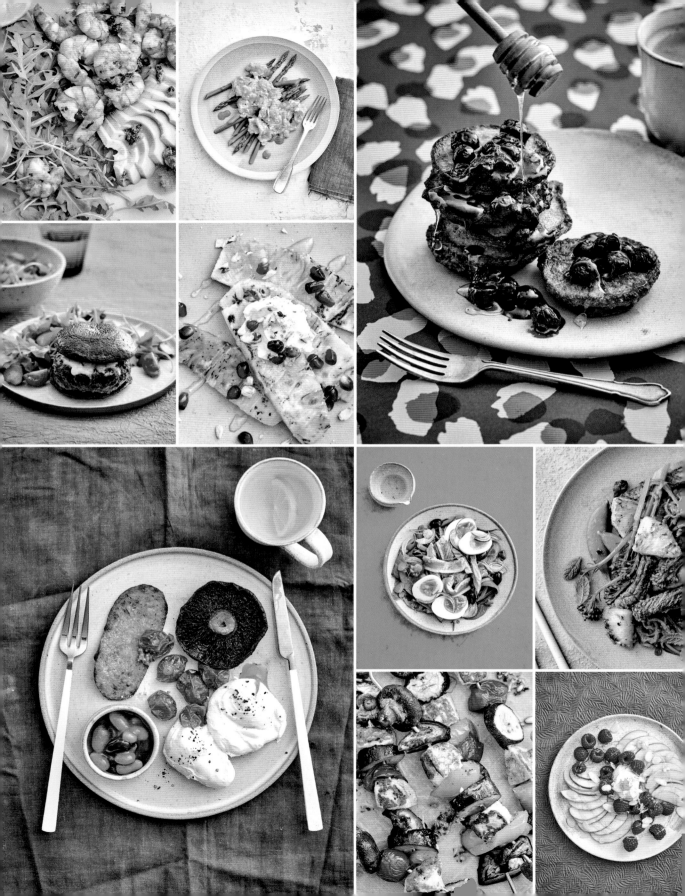

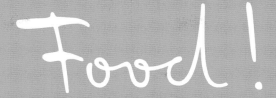

Food!

I've had it with
complicated meals that
take forever to make. I just
want to eat healthy fast
food, now!

- You'll have good food that's ready in as little as 15 minutes, so you can stay in shape even when life gets crazy.

- You'll cook with ingredients you can easily grab in the supermarket.

- I've sorted portion control and kept an eye on calories, so you don't have to stress.

- To help you get your 5-a-day in, each meal and snack contains fresh fruit or veg.

- You don't need fancy equipment.

- Every ingredient can be used in several different recipes, so nothing is wasted. Honestly, it drives me nuts when I have to buy one random ingredient and I don't know what to do with the rest of it. Supermarket superfoods are the way to go.

- Note: whenever I use eggs, I take them straight out the fridge and cook them from fridge-cold.

Breakfasts

HOW TO SHAPE UP
YOUR BREAKFAST

Eat before 10 o'clock – Maybe you're not a breakfast person. So if you don't fancy eating first thing in the morning, make life easy for yourself: grab a few healthy muffins (see page 35) to eat at your desk later. It not only saves you £4 buying takeaway every morning, but it means you won't attack and destroy the biscuit tin later because you're so ravenous.

Swap sugar for protein – There are a lot of eggs on the menu. Why? Protein-rich food, like eggs, means muscle repair and long-lasting energy for the day ahead. When I quit eating sugary cereals, I realised I started the day with a flatter belly, and I also had more energy.

Shake it off – I used to drink protein shakes after every workout. Protein shakes are helpful if you're lifting heavy weights, like I do sometimes. But if you're toning up with bodyweight workouts, as in this book, you're better off eating protein in actual food. I don't drink smoothies or juices either, as bought ones tend to have loads of sugar in them, while homemade ones are a faff to make and don't fill me up (so no smoothie recipes in this chapter! Soz).

Get fresh with me – I always have one piece of fresh fruit or veg with my breakfast.

Get caffeinated – First thing in the morning, a hot cup of black coffee with a tiny drop of honey wakes me right up. I find it helps with energy, digestion and metabolism straight away: all good for shaping up. It's also a great workout boost as the caffeine gets your muscles moving. I can't exercise on a full stomach, but as soon as my workout's done I'm excited for breakfast.

Say 'bye bye bread' – I don't keep bread in the house. If I have toast for breakfast I find that I'm hungry way before lunch. It's just not filling enough.

Mix it up – Try to mix up your breakfasts; it's healthier than eating the same thing every day. I'm not going to dictate exactly what to eat and when. Choose the foods that make you feel good and satisfy your appetite – some days you'll feel hungrier than others.

Do yourself a favour – Prep your breakfast the night before so you're not under pressure before work to cook anything. I don't have time to cook breakfast every morning, I don't expect you to either.

SIGNATURE EGGS ON ASPARAGUS

SERVES 1

Ready in 10 mins

1 tsp butter
50g asparagus (about 6
   spears)
2 medium eggs
½ tsp honey
salt and pepper
½ tsp piri piri sauce

If you're tired in the morning, this is for you. But you're going to have to trust me on this, OK? The secret ingredients are: honey and piri piri sauce. Just half a teaspoon of each with scrambled eggs is like magic. The sweet spiciness plus protein gives you serious get up and go.

Melt half the butter in a pan over a medium heat.

Break the woody ends off the asparagus and throw them away. Cook the asparagus for 5 minutes until they're buttery and glistening with some bite still.

Beat the eggs with a fork, then stir in the honey and a good grind of salt and pepper.

In a second pan (or put the cooked asparagus on a plate and use the same pan), melt the remaining butter over a medium heat. Scramble the eggs for 2–3 minutes, or until they are cooked how you like them.

Serve your eggs and asparagus with a dash of piri piri sauce.

THE VEGAN VERSION: Swap 1 tsp butter for 1 tsp olive oil; 2 eggs for 100g firm tofu, drained; and honey for maple syrup.

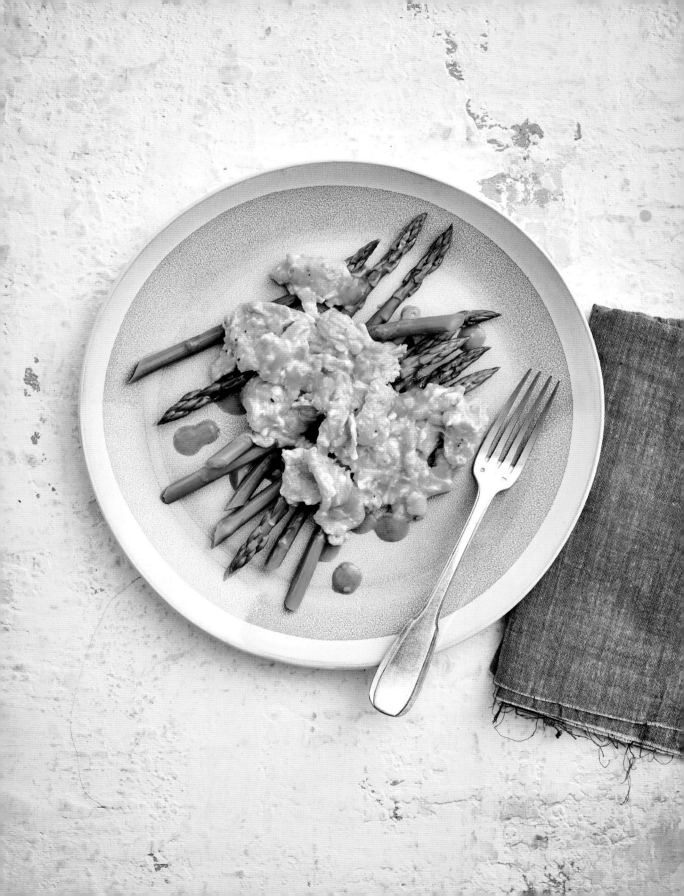

DIPPY EGGS WITH ASPARAGUS SOLDIERS

SERVES 1

Ready in 15 mins

1 tsp butter
50g asparagus (about 6
    spears)
2 medium eggs

I've been known to have a whole pack of asparagus with my dippy eggs, but asparagus is an expensive habit. Not as expensive as a handbag habit, but, you know. Try half a pack, or about six spears, and see how you get on. Warning: it is so tasty you'll probably want more.

Boil the kettle and pour the water into a pan over a medium heat. Bring the water back to the boil.

Melt the butter in a separate pan over a medium heat.

Break the woody ends off the asparagus and throw them away. Cook the asparagus for 5 minutes until they're buttery and glistening with some bite still.

Pop your eggs in the pan of boiling water. Put the lid on and boil them for 5 minutes (which should be just right for a dippy egg: the white sets and the yolk is runny. If you don't store your eggs in the fridge they'll cook a little faster).

Crack the top off your eggs, and dip in your asparagus soldiers.

FOLDED EGGS WITH SMOKED SALMON

SERVES 1

Ready in 15 mins

2 tsp butter
2 garlic cloves
50g mushrooms
30g kale
2 medium eggs
salt and pepper
50g smoked salmon

Like omelettes, but classier in my opinion. You can fill folded eggs with anything; I've gone for kale, mushrooms and smoked salmon, but red peppers, courgette and cheese would also work well.

Melt half your butter in a medium pan over a medium heat.

Grate your garlic straight into the pan. Slice your mushrooms and chuck them in.

Remove the stalks from your kale and throw them away. Chop the kale leaves up into easy to eat pieces.

Add the kale to the pan. Cook until the mushrooms are glistening and the kale's a tiny bit crunchy at the edges.

While the veg are cooking, melt the remaining butter in small non-stick pan over a medium heat.

Beat the eggs with a fork and add the salt and pepper.

Pour the eggs into the pan and use a spatula to fold the outside edge of the eggs in towards the middle, so the raw egg runs into the space. Keep folding for about a minute more, until the eggs are soft but no longer runny.

Serve your eggs like a calzone, filled with the hot kale and mushrooms and cold smoked salmon – which will warm through inside the eggs.

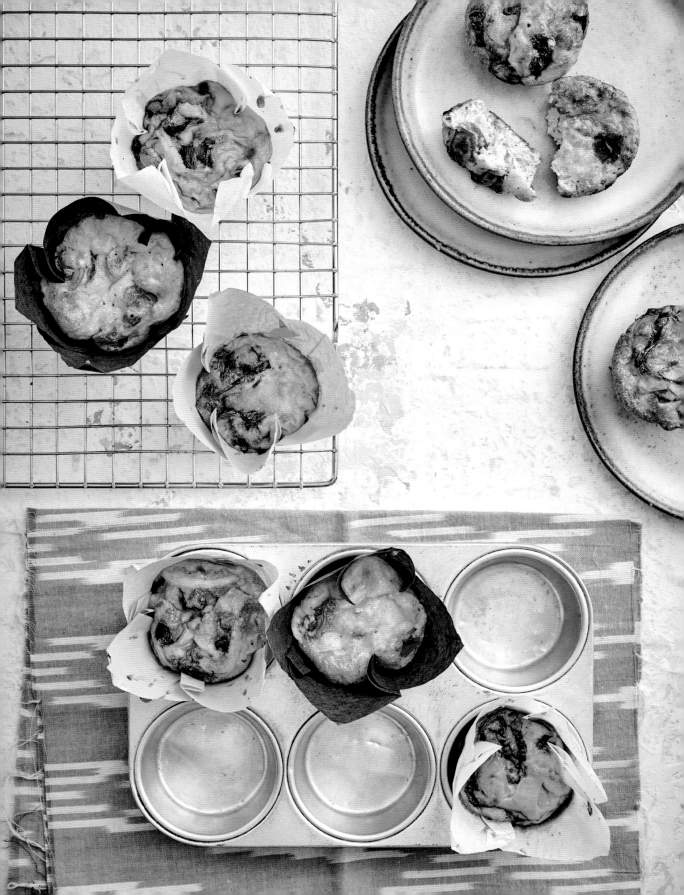

EGG MUFFINS

MAKES 12 MUFFINS,
OR 4–6 SERVINGS

Ready in 30 mins

8 medium eggs
½ tsp garlic salt
salt and pepper

**For smoked salmon and
spinach muffins:**

100g smoked salmon, sliced
into strips
1 big handful fresh spinach,
chopped

**For chicken and mushroom
muffins:**

100g pre-cooked chicken,
shredded
50g mushrooms, cut into
chunks

**For cheese and tomato
muffins:**

100g mature Cheddar,
grated
10 cherry tomatoes,
quartered

**Yum, these egg muffins are so gorgeous and poufy.
You can fill them with whatever you like, but I love
ingredients that don't need extra cooking first, like
smoked salmon, cheese, pre-cooked chicken, tomato,
mushroom and spinach. I'll have two for breakfast,
three if I'm really hungry. Store them in an airtight
container and they'll last up to 7 days in the fridge.**

Heat the oven to 200°C (or 180°C for a fan oven).

Grease and line 1 x 12-hole or 2 x 6-hole muffin tin(s). If
you're using paper muffin cases, double up to prevent leaks.

In a bowl, beat the eggs with a fork. Add your garlic salt
and salt and pepper, then the ingredients for your chosen
flavour, and give it a big stir.

Pour the mixture into your muffin tin so each hole is about
three-quarters full.

Bake for 20 minutes on the highest shelf of your oven
until the muffins have risen and are golden brown on top.
I usually go and have a shower while they're cooking and
come back to the kitchen when breakfast is ready.

If you're saving muffins for another time, give them a
chance to cool before you stash them away, otherwise
they'll go soggy. Who wants a soggy bottom in their life?

THE VEGAN VERSION: Swap 8 eggs for 300g firm tofu, drained
(your muffin looks less poufy, but still tastes good); salmon, chicken
or cheese for diced red pepper, grated courgette or frozen peas. If
you need something extra to bind the vegan ingredients together,
try 1 tbsp tahini.

HASH BROWN NEST

SERVES 1

Ready in 15 mins

½ sweet potato (about
    100g)
2 medium eggs
20g mature Cheddar
salt and pepper
¼ tsp dried chilli flakes
1 handful fresh baby spinach
6 cherry tomatoes, halved

Mmm, hash browns! Forget the processed, deep-fried kind found in greasy spoons; these sweet potato hash browns are the real deal. I love that moment when you break the yolk with your knife – yum-azing.

Heat the grill to high.

Peel and grate the raw sweet potato and squeeze out the excess liquid.

In a small bowl, beat one of your eggs. Grate in the cheese, then stir in salt, pepper and the chilli flakes, and then the grated sweet potato.

The messy bit: form the mixture into a rough circular mound and place on greaseproof paper on your grill pan. Use your fingers to mould the sweet potato into a nest shape: leave enough space to hold an egg inside.

Put under the grill.

After 5 minutes of cooking, remove the nest from the grill and crack the remaining egg into its centre. Put back under the grill until the white is set.

Serve with the baby spinach and cherry tomatoes.

THE VEGAN VERSION: Swap 2 eggs for 100g firm tofu (drained and crumbled) and place it in the centre of your sweet potato mixture; swap Cheddar for your favourite vegan cheese. If you need something extra to bind the sweet potato and vegan cheese, try 1 tbsp tahini.

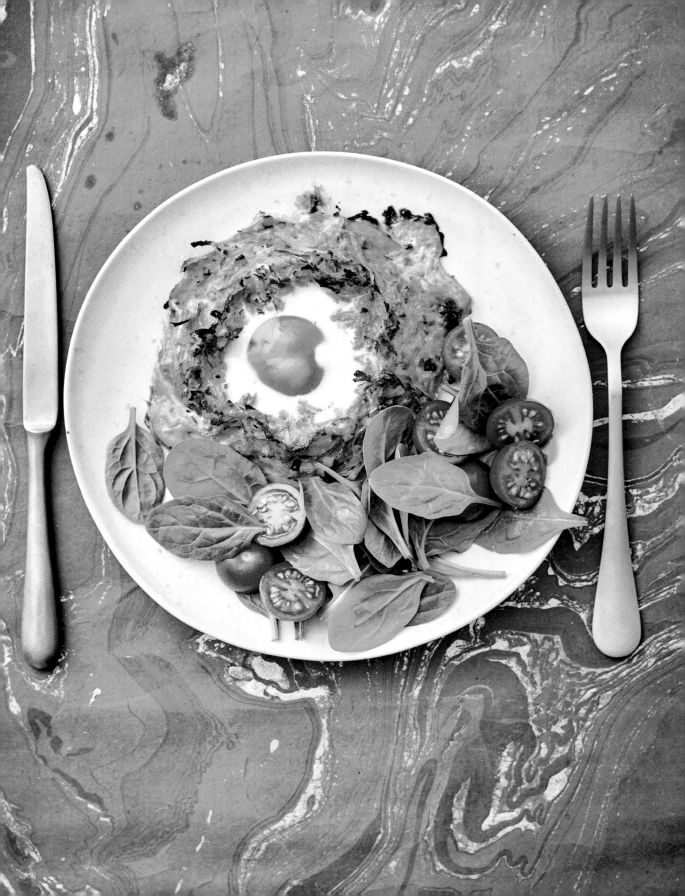

STUFFED PORTOBELLOS

SERVES 1

Mushrooms filled with flavour and topped with turkey bacon – yeees!

Ready in 20 mins

1 tsp butter
1 portobello mushroom
1 rasher turkey bacon
2 medium eggs
¼ tsp garlic powder
salt and pepper

Melt the butter in a large pan over a medium heat (or heat two medium-sized pans at the same time and divide up the butter – you can either fit everything in one large pan if you're careful the scrambled eggs won't run everywhere – you need to be on it with your spatula).

Pull the stalk off your portobello and pan-fry, whole, for 10 minutes, flipping after the first 5 minutes.

Add your turkey bacon to the pan, flipping regularly, for about 5 minutes. I like mine a bit crispy. Dab the cooked bacon with kitchen paper when it's done to remove the excess fat.

Beat your eggs with a fork, then stir in the garlic powder and salt and pepper. Scramble the eggs for 3–4 minutes, or until they are cooked how you like them.

Plate up the mushroom, top down, and pour the scrambled eggs over it, then balance your turkey bacon on top like a beret and tuck in.

THE VEGAN VERSION: Swap 1 tsp butter for 1 tsp olive oil; 2 eggs for 100g firm tofu (drained); and turkey bacon for vegan bacon.

SMOKY BEAN BOWL

SERVES 1

Ready in 15 mins

1 tsp butter
½ onion
1 garlic clove
100g mushrooms
1 rasher turkey bacon
1 tsp wholegrain mustard
¼ tsp smoked paprika
200g (½ can) baked beans
   – I love the kind with a mix
   of haricot, kidney, pinto,
   borlotti and cannellini
   beans (Heinz 5 Beanz is
   yum)
salt and pepper
2 medium eggs

You could faff about making your own beans, stirring passata and loads of pulses for hours. Or you could crack open a can of baked beans, stir in your smoky flavours and have brekkie on the table like, now. Hiding in the smoky loveliness are mushrooms and bacon, then layer two poached eggs on top to fire you up for the day.

Melt your butter in a pan over a medium heat.

Finely dice your onion and add it to the pan to soften for 5 minutes.

While the onion is softening, slice up your garlic, mushrooms and turkey bacon. Add them to the pan and cook for another 2 minutes.

Boil the kettle for the eggs.

Add the mustard, paprika and beans to the onion, bacon, garlic and mushrooms. Stir and add salt and pepper. Leave to gently cook while you poach your eggs.

To poach your eggs, fill a saucepan with about 5cm of boiling water, then lower the heat down to a simmer. One by one, crack each egg into a cup (this helps it slip into the pan), then stir the water to create a whirlpool and slide the egg into the middle. Cook for 3–4 minutes, or until the whites are set and the yolks are golden and runny. When the eggs are done, use a slotted spoon to lift them out and drain off the excess water.

Put the bean mixture in a bowl or lunchbox and serve the poached eggs on top.

THE VEGAN VERSION: Skip the eggs and turkey bacon; try topping with 2 rashers of vegan bacon instead; swap butter for olive oil.

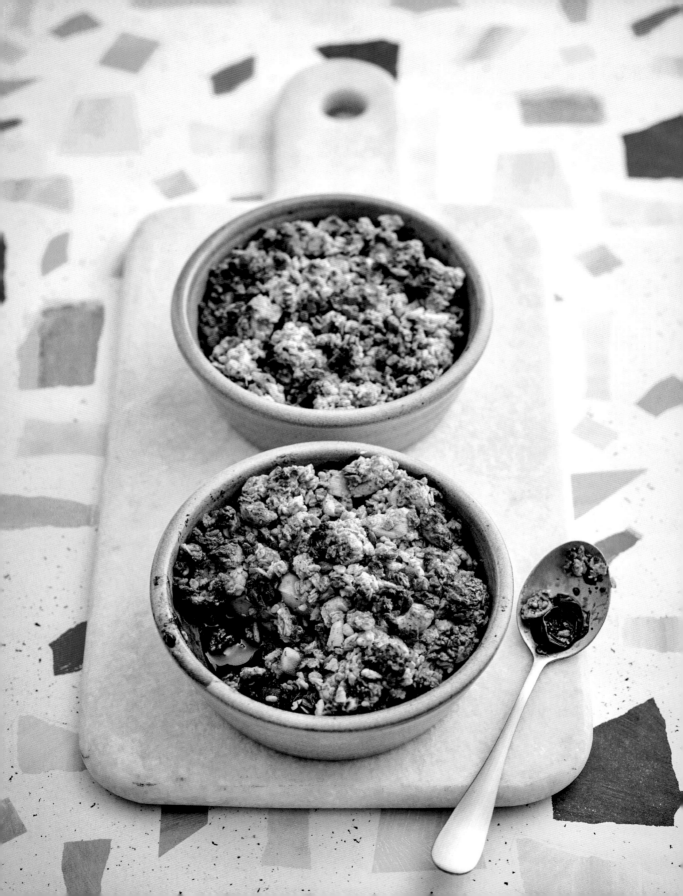

FRUIT AND NUT BAKE

MAKES 4 SERVINGS

Ready in 35 mins

100g pineapple or mango, peeled (if you only have canned pineapple, make sure it's in fruit juice, never syrup, with no added sugar)

3 eating apples (Pink Lady are my favourite)

200g blueberries (fresh or frozen)

60g unsalted cashew nuts

60g oats

2 tbsp unsweetened peanut butter

2 tbsp honey

1 tbsp butter

1 tsp vanilla extract

1 tsp freeze-dried raspberries (optional)

This cheeky crumble looks so impressive but is dead easy – imagine how heads will swivel in the office when you get this out at your desk. Bake these a couple of days before, then warm up your breakfast in the microwave when you get to work. I always used to make this with pineapple until I had an allergic reaction on holiday... So now I make it with mango. Both taste good!

Heat the oven to 200°C (or 180°C for a fan oven).

Core and dice the pineapple or mango and apples into small pieces and stir in your blueberries.

Chop your cashew nuts and chuck them in a bowl with the oats, peanut butter, honey, butter and vanilla extract. Use your hands to rub the ingredients together to evenly mix everything together and form the crumble.

Spoon the fruit mixture into a couple of ramekins, then layer the crumble on top.

Bake for 20 minutes, or until the apples are cooked through and the crumble is golden.

Sprinkle the freeze-dried raspberries on top to serve.

THE VEGAN VERSION: Swap 1 tbsp butter for 1 tbsp coconut oil and 2 tbsp honey for 2 tbsp maple syrup.

BANANA BLUEBERRY PANCAKES

SERVES 1

Ready in 15 mins

1 tsp butter
2 tbsp Greek yogurt
1 medium egg
50g oats
1 small ripe banana, peeled
1 tsp ground cinnamon
¼ tsp baking powder
50g blueberries (frozen or
  fresh)
1 drizzle honey (optional)

When I first tried blitzing banana and Greek yogurt for this recipe, I was like: Mind. Blown. So tasty and filling, with protein from both the egg and the yogurt. These only takes 15 minutes and are really filling so I have them for brunch as often as I fancy. Use frozen blueberries instead of fresh as they are cheaper to buy and last for ages in the freezer.

Melt the butter in a medium non-stick pan set over a medium heat.

Blend the rest of the ingredients together, saving the blueberries and honey for topping.

Pour palm-sized dollops of batter into the pan and cook for 2–3 minutes each side until golden.

In the last minute or two, add your frozen blueberries to the pan to heat them through. If you're using fresh blueberries, 30 seconds is enough to warm them up. I love it when my pancakes cook in the purple juice.

Stack your pancakes, top with the cooked blueberries and serve with a little drizzle of honey, if you fancy it.

THE VEGAN VERSION: Swap 1 tsp butter for 1 tsp coconut oil; 2 tbsp Greek yogurt for 2 tbsp soy yogurt; 1 egg for an extra ½ banana; 1 tbsp honey for 1 tbsp maple syrup. (This vegan version is lower in protein.)

Make a double batch of batter the night before to save time in the morning and the day after. It lasts up to 3 days, sealed in an airtight container in the fridge.

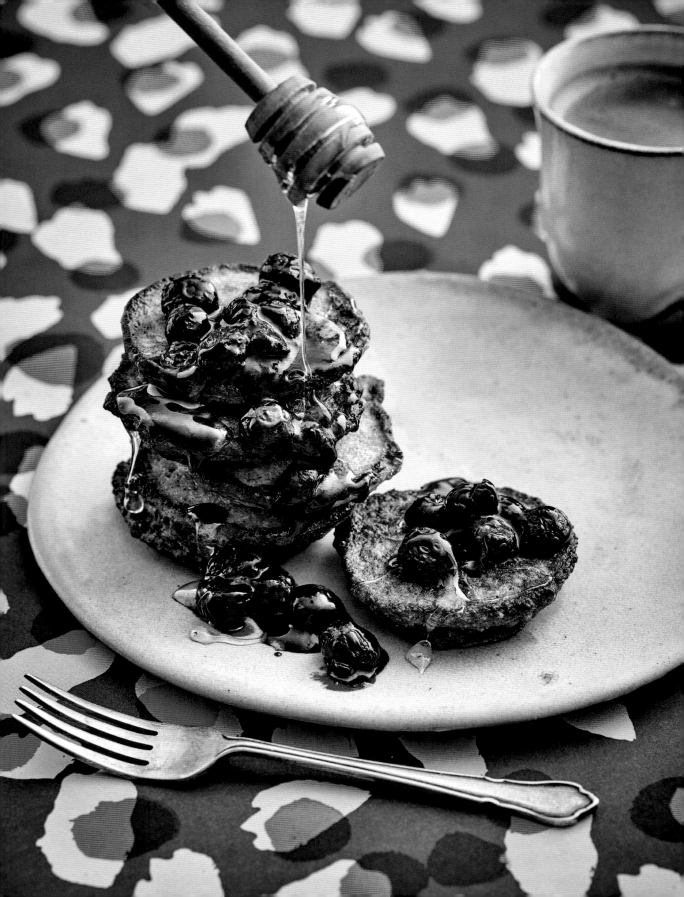

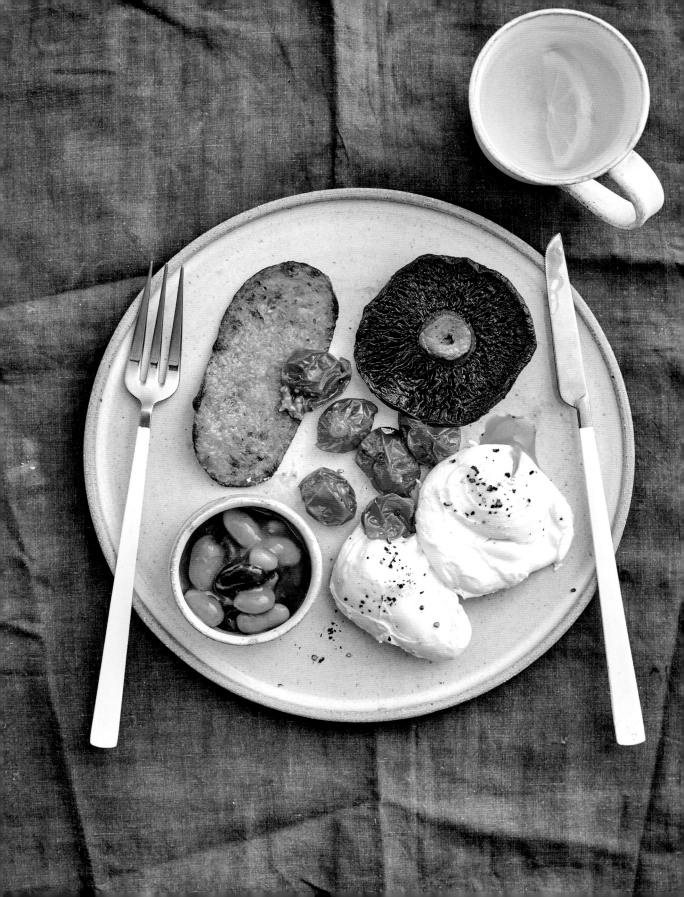

HALO FULL ENGLISH

SERVES 1

Ready in 15 mins

1 portobello mushroom
6 cherry tomatoes
salt and pepper
olive oil, to drizzle
1 rasher turkey bacon
1 tbsp baked beans (Heinz
    5 Beanz is good)
2 medium eggs

This protein-packed, low-carb, reduced-fat full English will help get you in shape for the day ahead and leave you feeling virtuous. What hangover?

Heat the grill to high.

Sprinkle your mushroom and tomatoes with salt and pepper and a tiny drizzle of olive oil.

Grill your turkey bacon, mushroom and tomatoes for about 10 minutes, turning every 2 or 3 minutes.

Put the baked beans in a little ovenproof ramekin and put under the grill too – it saves washing up a big pan. Just remember your oven gloves when you get it out, right?

In a different saucepan, poach your eggs. Fill the pan with about 5cm of boiling water, then lower the heat down to a simmer. One by one, crack each egg into a cup (this helps it slip into the pan), then stir the water to create a whirlpool and slide the egg into the middle. Cook for 3–4 minutes, or until the whites are set and the yolks are golden and runny. When the eggs are done, use a slotted spoon to lift them out and drain off the excess water.

Dab the cooked bacon with kitchen paper when it's done to remove the excess fat.

Plate it up with your mushroom, tomatoes, beans and eggs. Breakfast of champions.

Lunches

HOW TO SHAPE UP YOUR LUNCH

Think quick and easy – The best healthy lunch is one you can throw together super fast. It's so easy to make an amazing salad if you've got good ingredients ready to go, and if you prep lunch yourself, you can eat better food without spending a fortune. I cook with a lot of chicken, prawns and turkey mince because they're fantastic sources of lean protein and cook quickly.

Reinvent your leftovers – Last night it was chilli, today it's a wrap, a salad, a taco. Reworking your leftovers saves a ton of time and is so much more cost efficient. You'll find a few dinner recipes reincarnated as lunches here.

Plan your week ahead – Choose what you'd like for dinner, pick lunch recipes that rework those ingredients and batch cook. That means less time in the kitchen, and more time for you.

When are you working out today? If you go to the gym at lunchtime, bear in mind it's uncomfortable to do HIIT on a full stomach. Save lunch for after you shower. Every dish on the menu contains protein and healthy carbs (hello, veggies) to refuel after a workout and restore your body on rest days.

If you forget your lunchbox – go to the supermarket in your lunch break and grab a salad bag, tomatoes and an avocado, then top it with a cooked chicken breast, prawns, hard-boiled eggs or mackerel.

KING OF SALADS

SERVES 1

Ready in 10 mins

½ cooked beetroot
¼ red pepper, deseeded
6 cherry tomatoes
¼ cucumber
2 sticks celery
3 big handfuls salad, like spinach, watercress and rocket
50g stilton
150g cooked peeled king prawns
1 tbsp pomegranate seeds
1 dash piri piri sauce
juice of ¼ lemon

There's nothing worse than looking at a plate of salad and thinking, 'Where's the rest of it?' Enter the King Of Salads: my go-to. It's got so much going on that I always feel satisfied afterwards.

Chop your veggies, apart from your celery sticks, and toss them with the salad leaves.

Now, fill your celery sticks with the stilton, like canoes, and line your king prawns on top. Add to the salad and scatter with the pomegranate seeds. Treat yourself to a dash of piri piri sauce and a squeeze of lemon juice.

THE VEGAN VERSION: Swap 50g stilton for 50g hummus and 150g prawns for 150g mixed (canned) borlotti, flageolet and black beans.

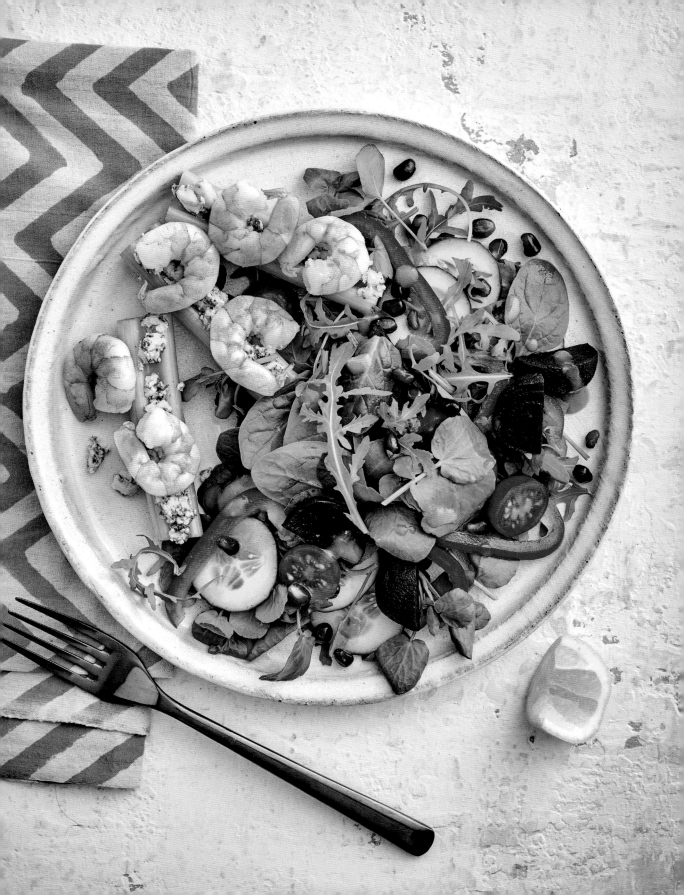

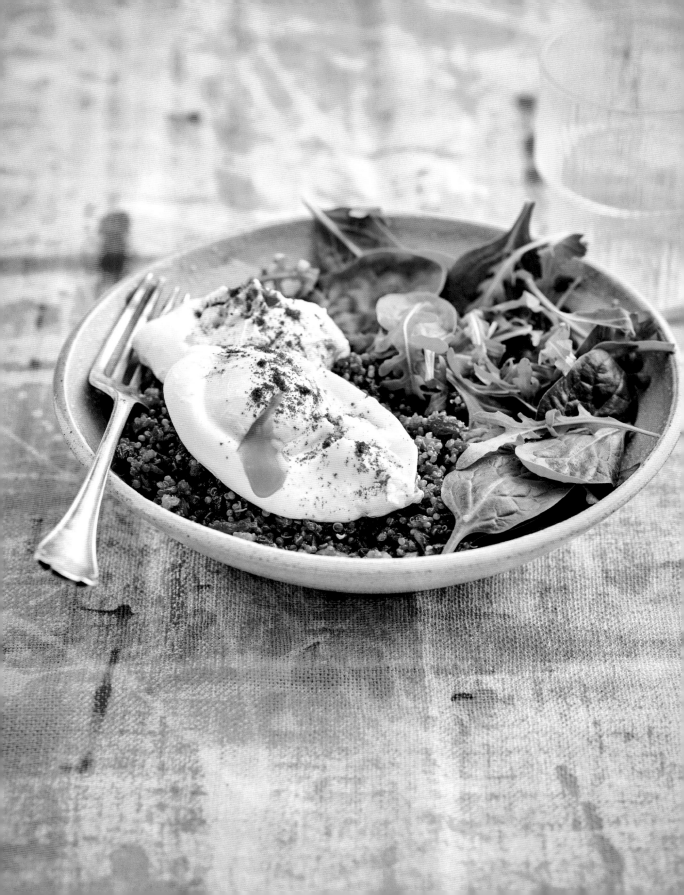

PINK QUINOA

SERVES 1

Ready in 15 mins

1 garlic clove
50g mushrooms
1 splash olive oil
100g cooked quinoa
1 tsp horseradish sauce
½ garlic salt
1 cooked beetroot
2 medium eggs
¼ tsp sweet paprika or dried
   chilli flakes, to serve
1 handful fresh spinach and
   rocket leaves, to serve

I'm a big fan of quinoa. Especially now I know how to pronounce it: keen-waa. Not only is it a great protein source, but you can load it up with flavour and it's a perfect pal for eggs.

Boil a kettle for your eggs.

Finely chop the garlic and slice the mushrooms.

Add a little olive oil to a pan over a medium heat.

Fry the garlic and mushrooms in the pan for 1 minute – if the garlic looks in danger of cooking too fast, turn down the heat.

Add the quinoa, horseradish and garlic salt.

Grate the beetroot straight into the pan. (Beetroot can stain your fingers, way worse than any fake tan, so I put clingfilm over my hand first.)

Cook everything together until hot.

While the quinoa mix is cooking, poach the eggs. Fill a saucepan with about 5cm of boiling water, then lower the heat down to a simmer. One by one, crack each egg into a cup (this helps it slip into the pan), then stir the water to create a whirlpool and slide the egg into the middle. Cook for 3–4 minutes, or until the whites are set and the yolks are golden and runny. When the eggs are done, use a slotted spoon to lift them out and drain off the excess water.

Put the pink quinoa into a bowl and top with the eggs. I sprinkle a tiny pinch of paprika or chilli flakes on top, and eat it with the spinach and rocket on the side.

THE VEGAN VERSION: Swap the eggs for extra veggies like ½ courgette and ¼ avocado, then add a generous dollop of hummus to bring it all together.

CLASSIC CHICKEN SALAD

SERVES 1

Grab all the ingredients from the supermarket on your lunch break and, boom! You're done.

Ready in 5 mins

1 cooked chicken breast
   (about 150g)
6 cherry tomatoes
¼ cucumber
¼ red pepper, deseeded
¼ red onion
¼ medium ripe avocado
3 big handfuls salad leaves,
   like spinach, rocket and
   watercress
1 handful pomegranate
   seeds
1 splash balsamic vinegar

Slice or tear the cooked chicken into bite-sized pieces.

Chop your veggies and avocado.

Arrange everything on a plate and sprinkle with the pomegranate seeds and a splash of balsamic vinegar. Grab yourself a fork and tuck in.

LEFTOVER BURRITOS

SERVES 1

Ready in 15 mins

1 portion last night's chilli
   (see page 88)
2 corn tortilla wraps
¼ avocado
1 handful fresh spinach
piri piri sauce (optional)

Give last night's chilli (see page 88) a makeover – those flavours will have really intensified. You can warm the chilli in the microwave at work if you want your wrap hot.

If you're taking this to work, box the chilli up separately from the fresh ingredients so the salad and wraps don't go soggy.

When you're ready to eat, warm the chilli and spoon it vertically into the tortilla wraps. Slice the avocado lengthways, then add the spinach and piri piri sauce if you want a bit of extra zing.

Roll up your wraps, tucking the ends in, and eat.

THE VEGAN VERSION: Swap turkey mince for the chilli for Quorn mince (see page 88).

SPICY STEAK WRAP

SERVES 1

Ready in 15 mins

150g leftover cooked steak
   (see page 93), chicken or
   lamb
½ gem lettuce
¼ avocado
¼ red pepper, deseeded
½ red chilli
20g cheese (extra-mature
   Cheddar or stilton gets
   my vote)
2 corn tortilla wraps
1 tbsp hoisin sauce
1 squeeze lemon juice

Do you ever cook a massive steak and think, 'I can't eat all that'? then eat it anyway, even though you're full? This is my favourite way to reinvent leftovers and make them stretch to an extra meal. This recipe also works with leftover cooked chicken or lamb – make use of whatever you've got.

Slice your meat, lettuce, avocado and red pepper. Remove the seeds from your chilli, unless you love your spice hot.

If you're using Cheddar, grate your cheese. If you prefer something like stilton, crumble it.

Soften each tortilla wrap by placing it in a hot dry frying pan for a minute.

Layer the meat, lettuce, avocado, red pepper, chilli and cheese into your tortilla wraps in a line down the middle. Add a dollop of hoisin, a good squeeze of lemon and roll them up ready to eat.

Wrap in foil and you're good to go.

THE VEGAN VERSION: Swap the meat for 100g cooked black beans and the dairy cheese for vegan cheese.

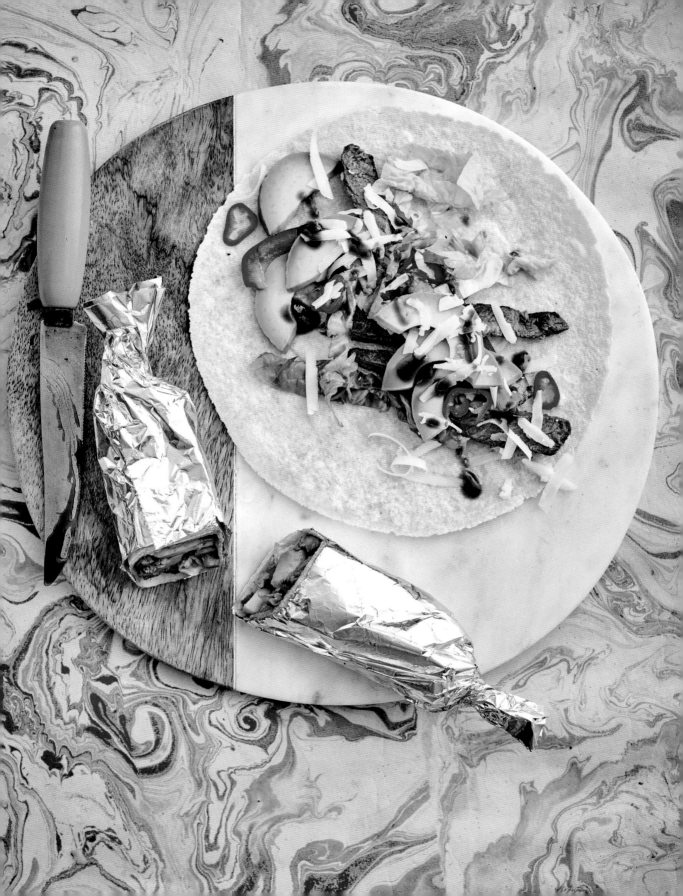

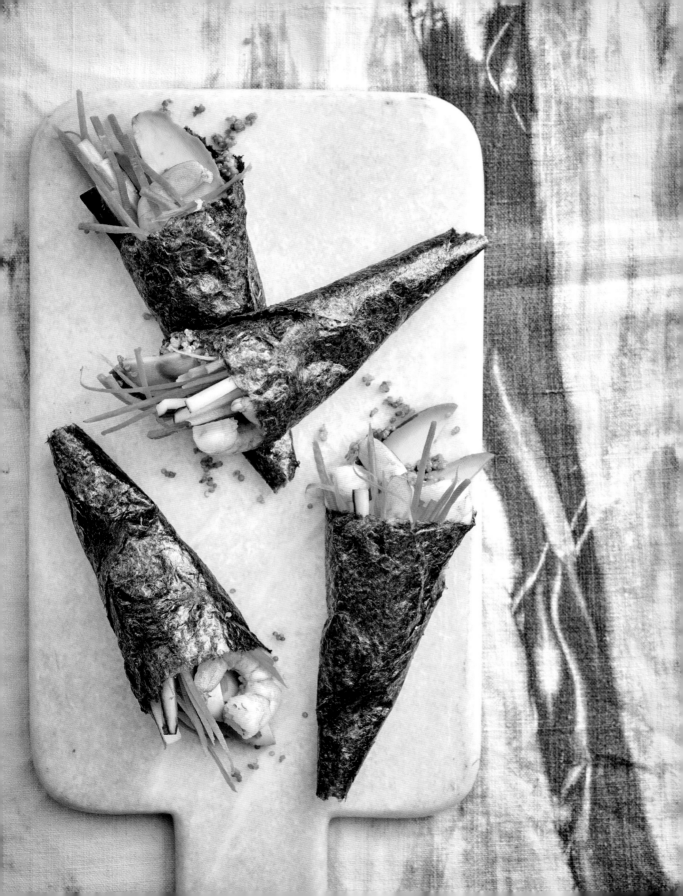

SUSHI WRAPS

SERVES 1

Ready in 10 mins

¼ avocado
¼ cucumber
¼ carrot
1 tbsp soy sauce (any kind),
   plus extra for dipping, if
   you wish
1 tsp fish sauce
1 tsp horseradish sauce (or
   wasabi)
1 tsp honey
50g cooked quinoa
100g cooked peeled prawns
4 nori seaweed sheets

I love sushi. This version's made with protein-rich quinoa instead of white rice. I also use horseradish to give these a kick because my local supermarket doesn't do wasabi, but use wasabi instead if you can get it.

Finely slice your avocado lengthways and chop the cucumber into matchsticks. Grate the carrot and squeeze its water out.

In a bowl, stir the sauces and honey into the cooked quinoa. It should be sticky, not wet, so drain off any excess liquid.

Spoon a quarter of your quinoa vertically on to a nori sheet, then add a quarter of your prawns, avocado and veg. Roll the nori into a cone. Repeat with the remaining ingredients to make four wraps.

FRIDGE MEZZE WITH FAST TZATZIKI

SERVES 1

Ready in 10 mins

For the tzatziki:
¼ cucumber
2 tbsp Greek yogurt
½ tsp dried chilli flakes
1 pinch salt
2 tsp mint sauce

Suggestions for your mezze:
50g cooked peeled prawns
50g cooked chicken
50g cooked mackerel
6 pitted black olives
50g sugarsnap peas
¼ red pepper, deseeded
6 cherry tomatoes
any leftover roast veg,
   such as sweet potato,
   aubergine, courgette or
   red onion

I love picky bits, and I especially love it when you can throw a gorgeous lunch together out of ingredients you just happen to have in the fridge. Pop it on a nice plate and ta-da! This super-fast tzatziki brings everything together.

To make the tzatziki, dice your cucumber, then stir it together with the other ingredients. Simple.

Chop everthing else into bite-sized pieces, arrange everything prettily on a big plate, then start dipping.

MACKEREL SUPER SLAW

SERVES 1

Ready in 10 mins

½ carrot

50g pickled red cabbage

1 tbsp Greek yogurt

1 tsp mustard (grainy or
    Dijon works: pick your
    favourite)

salt and pepper

6 cherry tomatoes

¼ cucumber

2 big handfuls spinach,
    watercress and rocket
    salad

150g cooked mackerel, skin
    removed

1 lemon wedge

Mackerel is every fit foodie's best-kept secret. It's a great source of protein and the kind of healthy fats that make your skin glow. You can get mackerel ready-cooked from the supermarket and make a salad in no time at all.

To make your slaw, grate the carrot and mix it with the red cabbage, yogurt and mustard. Season well. If you're taking this to work, seal the slaw in a separate box.

Halve the cherry tomatoes and cut the cucumber into bite-sized pieces.

Arrange your salad leaves, tomatoes and cucumber in your lunchbox, then lay your mackerel on top. Have a lemon wedge ready to spritz over your fish just before eating.

STUFFED PEPPERS

SERVES 1

Ready in 60 mins

1 red or yellow pepper
2 garlic cloves
6 mushrooms
salt and pepper
1 drizzle olive oil
1 tsp butter
1 rasher turkey bacon
2 medium eggs
6 pitted black olives
6 cherry tomatoes
½ tsp dried Italian herbs, like
    oregano or basil
2 big handfuls spinach,
    watercress and rocket
    salad
1 splash balsamic vinegar

I love a hollow pepper; you can fill them with anything. I've gone for scrambled egg, mushrooms, bacon and black olives here, but you can also try cheese, smoked salmon, avocado... whatever floats your boat. You can roast the pepper a day in advance, or chuck it in the oven before a workout. Get your sweat on, then eat.

Heat the oven to 160°C (or 140°C for a fan oven).

Slice the pepper in half lengthways and deseed. Peel and halve the garlic cloves. Quarter the mushrooms.

Divide the garlic and mushrooms between your pepper halves, then season with salt and pepper.

Give them a quick drizzle of olive oil before sliding the filled pepper halves into the oven on a greased baking tray.

Roast for 50–60 minutes while you work out.

In the last 5 minutes of cooking time (you can leave your pepper in the still-warm oven if you've done a long workout), melt the butter in a nice big pan over a medium heat.

Cut the turkey bacon into strips and cook for 3–4 minutes, then add your eggs to scramble, along with the olives and tomatoes.

Scatter the herbs over the whole lot.

Take the peppers out of the oven and plate up. Fill each half with the scrambled egg mix and serve with the salad leaves and a good splash of balsamic.

Save time: Put extra filled peppers in the oven to roast and have them ready in the fridge to eat for lunch tomorrow or another night's dinner later in the week.

THE VEGAN VERSION: Swap butter for olive oil; 2 eggs for 100g firm tofu (drained, then scrambled); turkey bacon for vegan bacon.

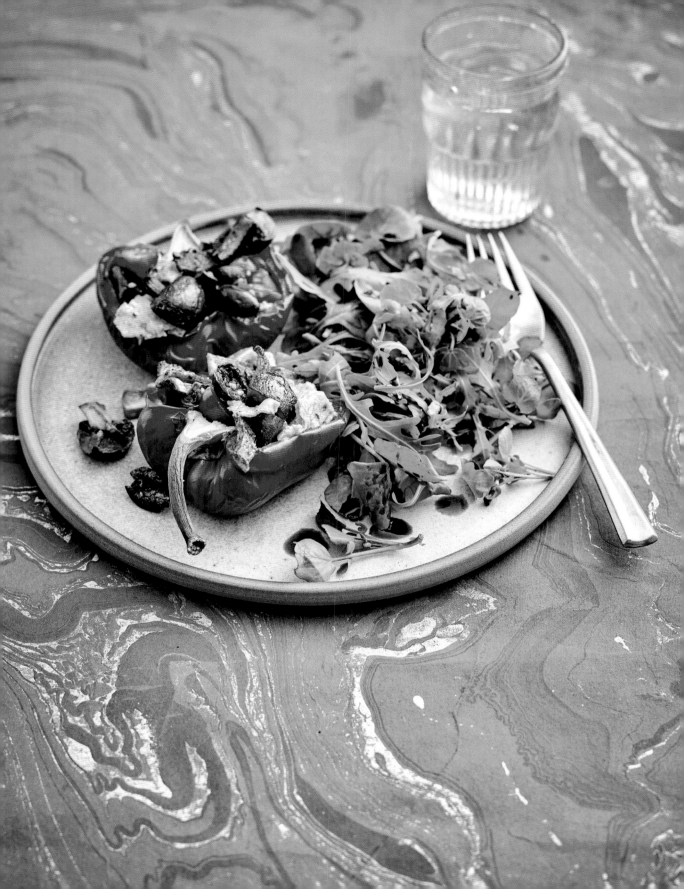

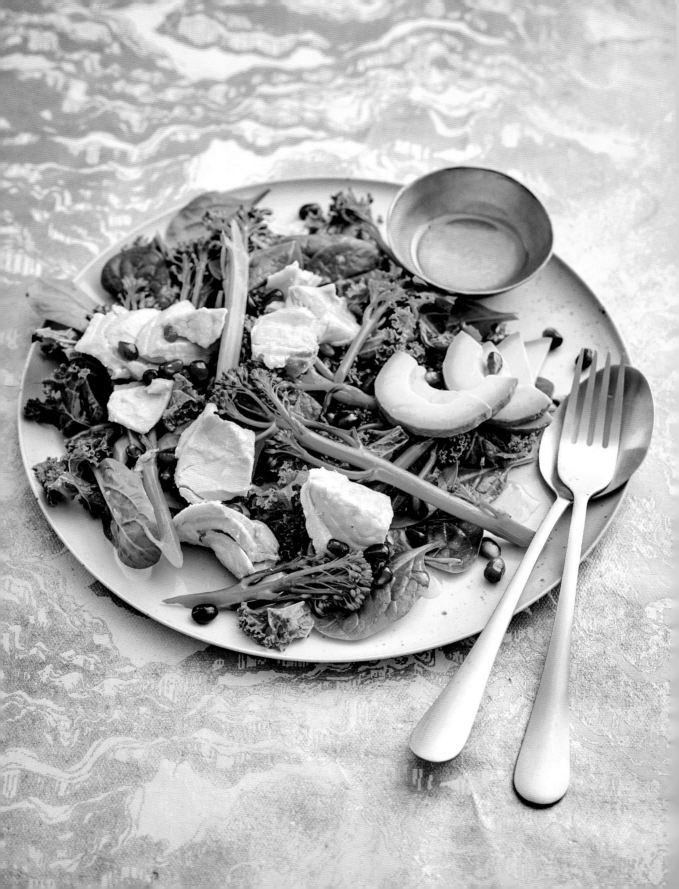

SALMON SUPERFOOD SALAD

SERVES 1

Ready in 15 mins

100g tenderstem broccoli
50g kale
juice of ½ lemon
¼ avocado
150g cooked salmon fillet
50g baby spinach leaves
1 tbsp pomegranate seeds

For the zesty lemon dressing:
zest and juice of ½ lemon
1 pinch salt
2 tsp olive oil

Show me a superfood and I'm interested. Show me a whole giant salad packed with an all-star line-up of superfoods and drizzled with zesty lemon dressing, and I'm grabbing a fork.

Boil the kettle and put the water in a pan over a high heat.

Add the broccoli to the pan and simmer for 3–4 minutes, or until just tender.

Remove the stalks from your kale and throw them away. Chop the kale leaves up into easy to eat pieces.

Rub the lemon juice into the kale to soften the leaves and leave for a couple of minutes while you make the dressing.

Whip up your dressing: use a grater to zest the lemon, then mix it with the juice, salt and olive oil. Set aside.

Slice your avocado and flake the salmon.

Mix the baby spinach leaves with the kale and plate up with the broccoli.

Top with the avocado and salmon. Scatter with the pomegranate seeds and pour over the dressing.

If you're taking this to work, pack your dressing in a separate tiny pot so your leaves stay nice and fresh.

BEST TUNA NIÇOISE

SERVES 1, PLUS
LEFTOVERS

Ready in 15 mins

2 medium eggs
60g green beans
¼ red onion
6 cherry tomatoes
½ salad bag of spinach,
    watercress and rocket
    leaves
6 pitted black olives
150g tuna, either leftover
    cooked tuna steak or
    canned (see page 86 for
    cooking method)

For the dressing:
½ tsp mustard
juice of ¼ lemon
1 tsp olive oil
salt and pepper

Why is it the best? Because it's made with leftover seared tuna steak – my favourite. You can use canned tuna, if you prefer; you're making this salad for you! It's the extras like black olives, sticky hard-boiled eggs and green beans that make this salad a showstopper. Customise this recipe however you like: add anchovies for a classic niçoise, or if you have leftover sweet potato wedges they'd taste great too.

Boil the kettle. Put the water in a pan over a medium heat.

Add the eggs to the pan and boil for 7 minutes, so they're firm but the yolks are still sticky.

After the first 2 minutes of cooking, top and tail your green beans and add them to the egg pan. Boil for 4–5 minutes.

Drain the eggs and beans; put the boiled eggs in a bowl of cold water to stop them going too hard.

Finely slice the red onion and halve the tomatoes. Lay out your bed of salad leaves and add your cooked and raw veggies, olives and sliced cooked tuna (or flaked canned tuna).

Peel and halve the eggs and arrange on top.

Make the dressing: stir the mustard, lemon juice, olive oil and seasoning together. Drizzle over the salad.

This salad works warm or cold, so you can box it up or eat right now. If you do take it to work, carry your dressing in a little pot so your salad leaves stay fresh.

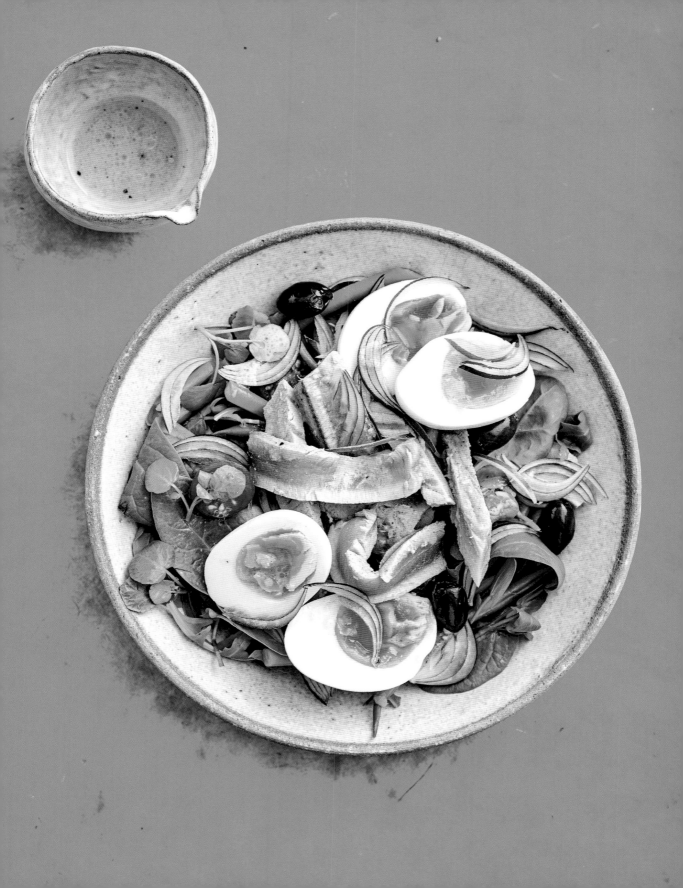

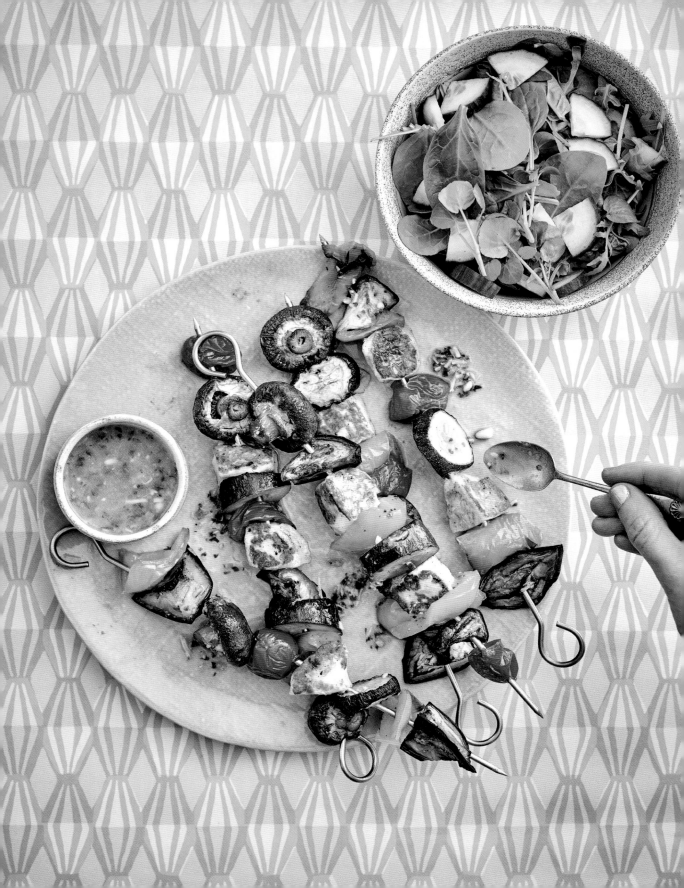

ZINGY VEG SKEWERS

SERVES 1

Ready in 60 mins

½ aubergine
1 yellow pepper, deseeded
½ courgette
1 drizzle olive oil
salt and pepper
125g halloumi
6 mushrooms
6 cherry tomatoes
2 big handfuls mixed salad
　　leaves, such as spinach,
　　watercress and rocket
¼ cucumber, sliced

For the dressing:
1 tbsp pesto
zest and juice of 1 lemon

Such a gorgeous, sunny dish. You can make these skewers with leftover roast vegetables from your meal prep frenzy and mix in fresh salad veggies too. The zingy dressing brings it all together.

Heat the oven to 200˚C (or 180˚C for a fan oven).

Chop your aubergine, pepper and courgette into chunks, then spread them all out in a roasting tin, and treat them to a good drizzle of olive oil, plus salt and pepper. Place them in the oven to roast.

Cube the halloumi and set aside.

When the veggies have been roasting for about 20 minutes, remove the tin from the oven.

Skewer the aubergine, pepper and courgette chunks with the mushrooms, tomatoes and halloumi cubes. (Keep the mushrooms and tomatoes whole to make skewering easier.)

Place the skewers in the roasting tin, return to the oven and roast everything for another 20 minutes.

Just before your skewers are ready, mix the pesto with the lemon zest and juice to make the dressing. Give it a good grind of salt and pepper.

Scatter the salad leaves with the cucumber, serve with the skewers and be generous with the dressing.

THE VEGAN VERSION: Swap the halloumi for skewered cauliflower florets.

These kebabs are a great one to chuck on the barbecue too – give them up to an hour on the grill, or until hot and nicely charred, and remember to keep turning the skewers. Drizzle over the dressing once barbecued.

RAINBOW SALAD

SERVES 1

Ready in 60 mins

125g halloumi
½ sweet potato
1 red onion
½ aubergine
olive oil, to drizzle
dried rosemary, to sprinkle
1 courgette
1 yellow pepper, deseeded
6 cherry tomatoes
¼ cucumber, sliced
6 pitted black olives
2 handfuls mixed salad
    leaves like spinach,
    watercress and rocket

**For the pomegranate
    dressing:**

1 tbsp pomegranate seeds
2 tsp balsamic vinegar
1 tsp olive oil
salt and pepper

This is a masterclass in how meal prep makes your life easy. Every single ingredient can either be cooked or prepped up to 3 days ahead of time so you can grab and go from the fridge. The prep takes about 1 hour, the assembly takes about 5 minutes!

The get-ahead part:

Heat the oven to 180°C (or 160°C for a fan oven).

Cut the halloumi into thick slices and fry in a dry pan or on a griddle until golden. Cool and keep in the fridge until needed. Dice up the cold halloumi when you are ready to make the salad.

Chop the sweet potato, onion and aubergine into wedges and arrange on a roasting tray, drizzled with olive oil and sprinkled with dried rosemary. Roast in the oven for about 50 minutes until soft and golden. Leave to cool and keep in the fridge in an airtight container.

Chop the courgette into rounds and slice the pepper and arrange on a roasting tray with the tomatoes. Drizzle with olive oil and roast for about 30 minutes, or until softened and golden. Leave to cool and keep in the fridge in an airtight container.

The fast assembly part:

If you fancy a warm salad you can heat the roast veg and halloumi gently under the grill or in the microwave, minus the leaves and cucumber.

Otherwise, plate up the fresh ingredients: cucumber, olives and salad leaves. Top with the rainbow of roast veg and halloumi.

Stir the dressing ingredients together, then pour over the salad just before you want to eat.

THE VEGAN VERSION: Swap the halloumi for griddled cauliflower wedges.

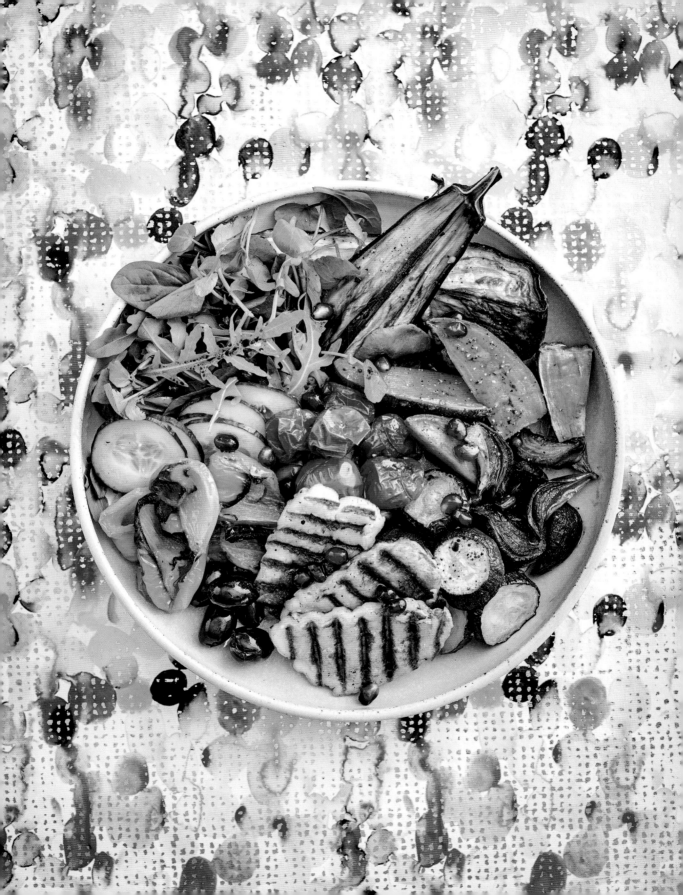

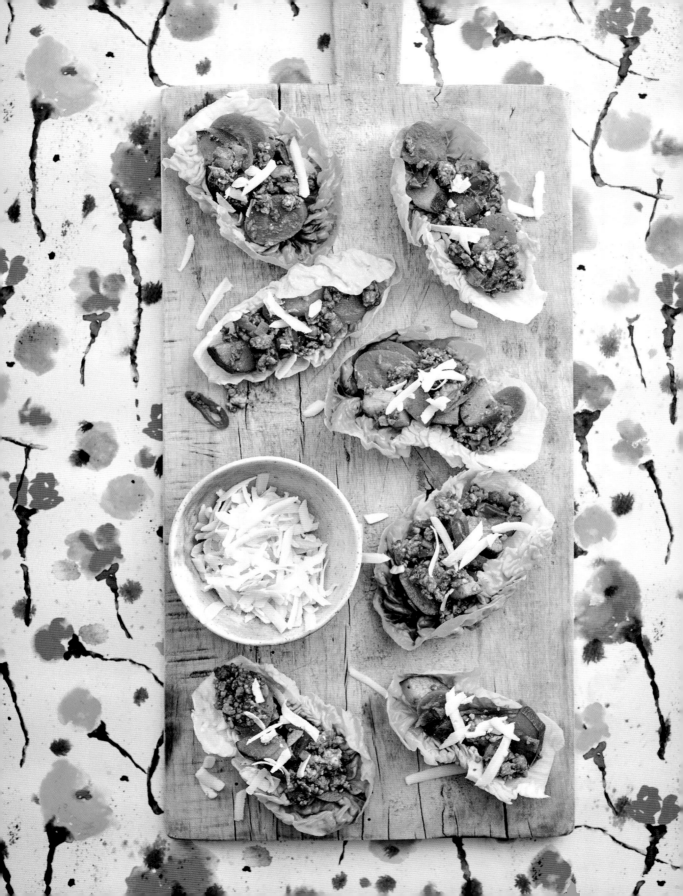

GREEN TACOS

<table>
<tr><td>SERVES 1</td></tr>
</table>

Ready in 15 mins

1 gem lettuce
1 portion last night's chilli
  (see page 88)
20g Cheddar cheese, grated
dried chilli flakes (optional)

Look, I know this recipe seems like a bit of a cheat, but why not make life easy? You're going to make green tacos with leftover chilli – green because Mother Nature has conveniently grown a gem lettuce into just the right shape.

Separate the leaves of your lettuce. Heat up last night's chilli, then load up each 'taco' leaf.

Add a sprinkle of grated cheese and some chilli flakes, if you fancy.

Eat.

THE VEGAN VERSION: Swap turkey mince for the chilli for Quorn mince and Cheddar for vegan cheese.

PAPRIKA PRAWNS WITH THREE GREENS

SERVES 1

Ready in 15 mins

2cm-piece fresh ginger
¼ tsp paprika
juice of ½ lime
150g raw tiger prawns,
    peeled
100g broccoli
100g sugarsnap peas
2 large handfuls kale
2 tsp sesame or vegetable
    oil
1 tbsp pomegranate seeds

This one's delicious hot or cold. I've gone for cooked greens in this recipe, but you could go for fresh: avocado, spinach, watercress. Raw sugarsnaps work well too. Add an easy dressing, like the zesty lemon number on page 63, if you fancy.

Peel and grate the fresh ginger. Mix together with the paprika and lime juice and then tip in the prawns and leave them to marinate.

Chop the broccoli into small pieces. Cook with the sugarsnap peas in a pan of boiling salted water for 3–4 minutes until just tender.

Remove the stalks from your kale and throw them away. Chop the kale leaves up into easy to eat pieces. Add them to the broccoli pan for the last minute of cooking. Drain all the veg.

Heat the oil in a second pan over a high heat and cook the marinated prawns until they turn pink. Add the marinade to the prawns and cook for 30 seconds.

Toss everything together and serve with the pomegranate seeds sprinkled on top.

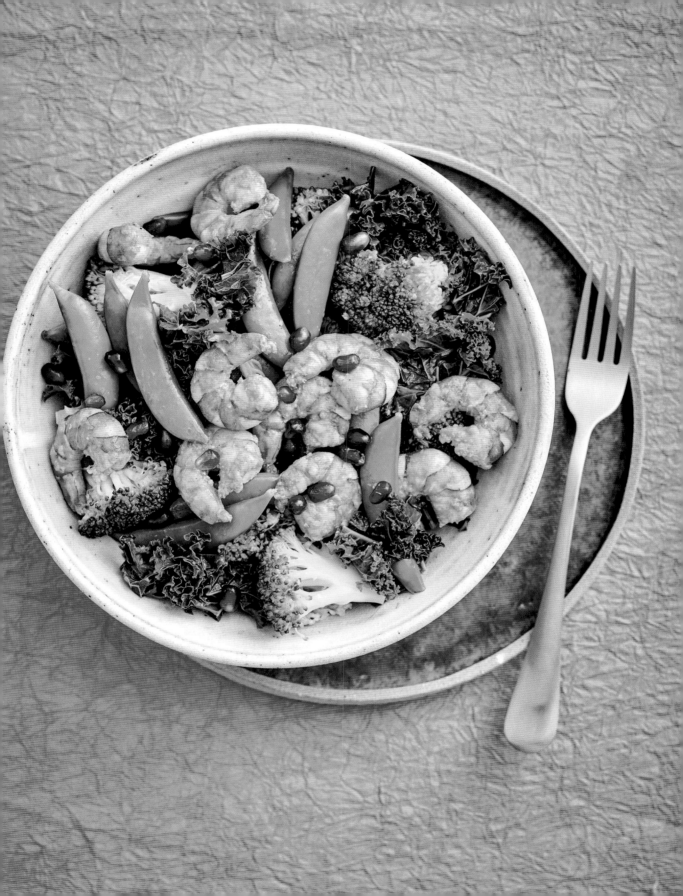

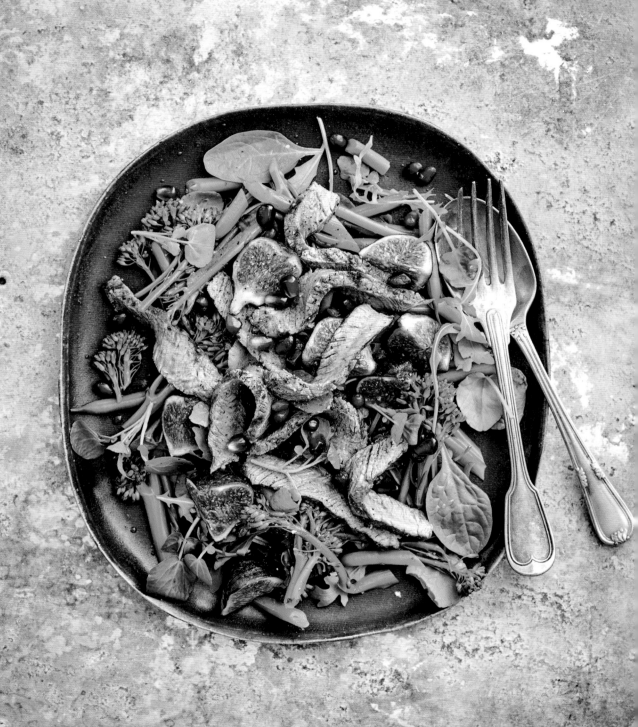

STEAK AND FIG SALAD

SERVES 1

Ready in 10 mins

100g cooked steak (see
   page 93)
2 fresh figs
50g green beans
50g tenderstem broccoli
salt and pepper
½ salad bag of mixed
   spinach, watercress and
   rocket
1 tsp pomegranate seeds
1 drizzle olive oil
juice of ¼ lemon

There's something about salty steak paired with sweet figs. Perfect partners. Last night's steak gets a whole new lease of life. If you polished off your green beans and tenderstem broccoli last night, they cook in less than 5 minutes, so you can totally make this work.

Slice your cooked steak into strips, quarter the figs and chop the veg into bite-sized chunks.

Cook the beans and broccoli pieces in a pan of boiling salted water for about 2 minutes, or until just tender, then drain.

Arrange the veg on a bed of green leaves, top with the steak strips and fig quarters and scatter with the pomegranate seeds. Grind over some salt and pepper and drizzle with olive oil and lemon juice.

ROAST LAMB WITH ALL THE TRIMMINGS

SERVES 2,
PLUS LEFTOVERS

Ready in 3 hours 30 mins

3 garlic cloves
1 tbsp olive oil
salt and pepper
1 tsp dried oregano
1 tsp dried rosemary
1 small rolled shoulder
   of lamb (about 500g –
   aim for 150g per person,
   allowing you 150g for
   a leftovers lunch)
3 sweet potatoes
3 carrots
½ mug stock (optional)
1 onion
1 splash balsamic vinegar
Bisto, to taste (optional)
100g pickled red cabbage
1 head broccoli
5 big handfuls kale
4 tbsp frozen peas
2 tsp mint sauce, to serve

You know you're officially a grown-up when you do a roast... I used to be a bit scared of cooking a roast, but recently my boyfriend and I did it together and it was insane. It'll make your Sunday sing and set you up for a great week because you've got tons of healthy leftovers to use in other dishes.

Heat the oven to 180°C (or 160°C for a fan oven).

Peel and grate the garlic, then mix it with the olive oil, seasoning and herbs. Rub this over the lamb, getting your hands right in there, then place in a roasting tray.

Peel and chop the sweet potatoes and carrots into chunks and arrange them around the meat so they cook in the juices. Cover with foil and roast for 2–3 hours, depending on the size of your joint – you've got a great workout window here if you want it!

Check back periodically to spoon fat from the roasting tray over the lamb. Once cooked, take the meat out of the oven and leave to rest for at least 20 minutes, covered in foil.

While the meat is resting, make your gravy. The easy way is to add 2 tablespoons hot lamb fat to ½ mug stock. Or, I like to make caramelised onion gravy, which is chunkier. Slice the onion, then gently cook in a small saucepan with 2 tablespoons hot lamb fat from the roasting tray. Keep the heat low, add a good splash of balsamic vinegar and let the onion caramelise. Cook it slowly for 10 minutes, stirring occasionally. Put it in a bowl ready to serve. (You could add some Bisto in to make this more gravy-like too, although it adds more calories.)

Spoon your pickled red cabbage into a small baking dish and leave in the still-warm oven to heat through.

Chop up the broccoli and cook in boiling salted water for about 10 minutes, adding the kale (stalks removed; leaves chopped) and frozen peas for the last 3–4 minutes of time.

Serve it all up. Yum.

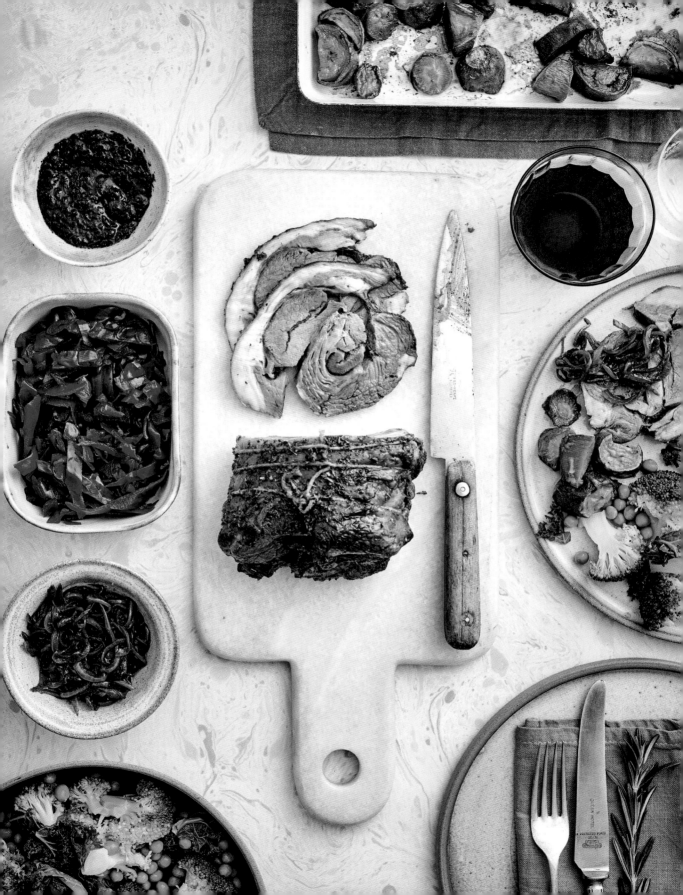

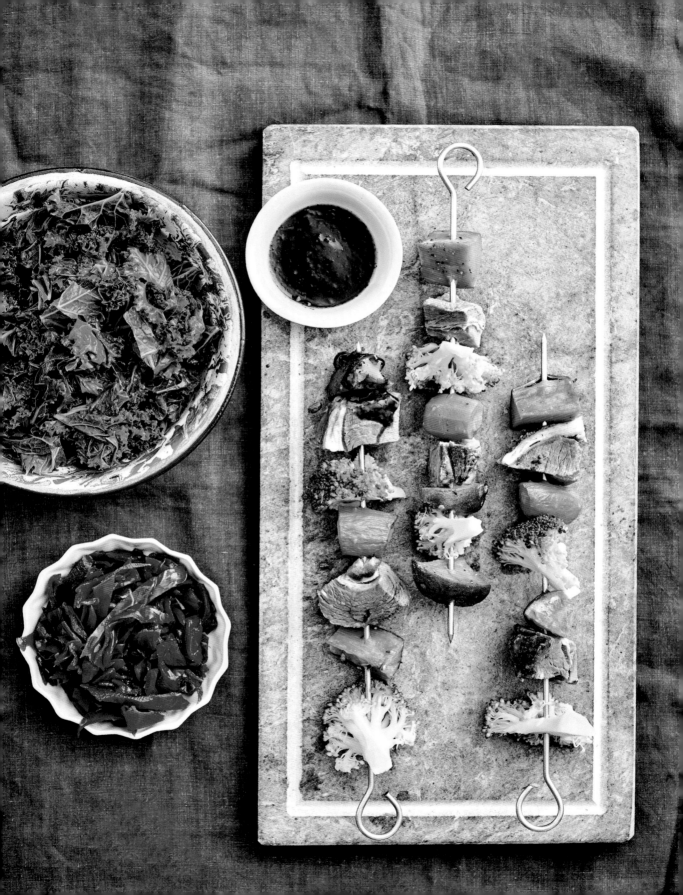

LEFTOVER LAMB WITH HOT MINT DIP

SERVES 1

Ready in 10 mins

150g cooked lamb (beef or
    chicken also work well if
    you prefer), diced
250g leftover roast veg
50g pickled red cabbage
handful of kale

For the dip:
1 tsp hot pepper sauce
1 tsp mint sauce
1 tsp balsamic vinegar

Mondays are hard enough without the old, 'What's for lunch?' dilemma. This is where your Sunday roast saves your ass. I've made you a spicy hot mint dip here to add some zing to your leftovers.

Dice the meat into chunks.

Mix the cold meat and veggies together on a plate or in your lunchbox. Or, thread on to metal skewers and put under the grill until piping hot – about 15 minutes.

Stir the dip ingredients together and either drizzle over your salad or put in a small bowl ready to dunk the skewers into.

Serve with the sides of red cabbage and kale. Hey presto! Roast, reinvented.

THE VEGAN VERSION: Swap 150g meat for 2 portobello mushrooms and add an extra dip of 2 tbsp hummus. It's lower in protein, but still delicious.

PEA AND PRAWN SALAD BOX

SERVES 1

Ready in 15 mins

5 cornichons
¼ medium avocado
½ baby gem lettuce
1 pinch fresh mint leaves
150g cooked peeled king
    prawns
4 tbsp cooked peas

For the dressing:
1 tsp mint sauce
1 tsp olive oil
1 tsp mustard (grainy or
    Dijon both work)
juice of ¼ lemon
salt and pepper

I had something like this when I was out for dinner somewhere posh, and I was like, wow, I want to eat this gorgeousness every day for the rest of my life. Only a tiny exaggeration. But here it is: one beautiful salad box. I love those little gherkins, they really pack a punch, flavour-wise.

Slice the cornichons and avocado, then shred the lettuce and finely chop the mint.

Add in the prawns and peas, and give the salad a big old toss together.

Mix the dressing ingredients together and pour over the salad right before you eat.

GREEN QUEEN CHICKEN STIR-FRY

SERVES 1

Ready in 10 mins

1 cooked chicken breast
　　or 150g cooked peeled
　　prawns
1 lunchbox full of stir-fried
　　veggies
1 handful fresh spinach
¼ avocado
juice of ½ lemon
salt and pepper
dried chilli flakes (optional)

This is a pure leftovers recipe using cooked chicken or prawns and stir-fried veg (add extra veg to the wok when you're making the recipes on pages 101 or 103). Green beans, tenderstem broccoli, kale, courgettes, sugarsnap peas, asparagus, get them all in there.

Slice or tear up the chicken, if using. Add the chicken or prawns, the cooked veggies, spinach and avocado to a lunchbox or plate up.

Squeeze over the lemon juice and season with salt and pepper, and chilli flakes, if you fancy. Done.

NO LEFTOVERS? If you don't have leftovers but want to make this recipe, stir-fry the chicken/prawns and veggies in a little hot oil for about 5 minutes until cooked. Add in the rest of the ingredients and tuck in.

Dinners

HOW TO SHAPE UP YOUR DINNER

Find a workout window – When I exercise in the evening, I'll take 5–10 minutes to prep dinner and put it in the oven so it's ready after my workout.

Know yourself – If you know you'll get in from work and you need to eat RIGHT NOW THIS SECOND, stock your fridge with ingredients from this book. OK, it's not technically NOW but you can hang on for 15 minutes.

Eat the essentials – My dinner essentials are protein + healthy carbs + flavour + just the right amount of fat to feel satisfied. I prefer a hot meal as it's more filling and easier to digest.

Go large – I'm always hungrier at the end of the day, so I have my biggest meal in the evening. I used to try and have something light, but that basically meant I'd go back to the fridge when dinner was over because I can't go to bed hungry. So: it's healthier to go with your feelings. You know you.

If you need an extra something... Enjoy it. I usually have one snack during the day and save a little dessert fix for after dinner – see my favourite recipes on pages 118–135.

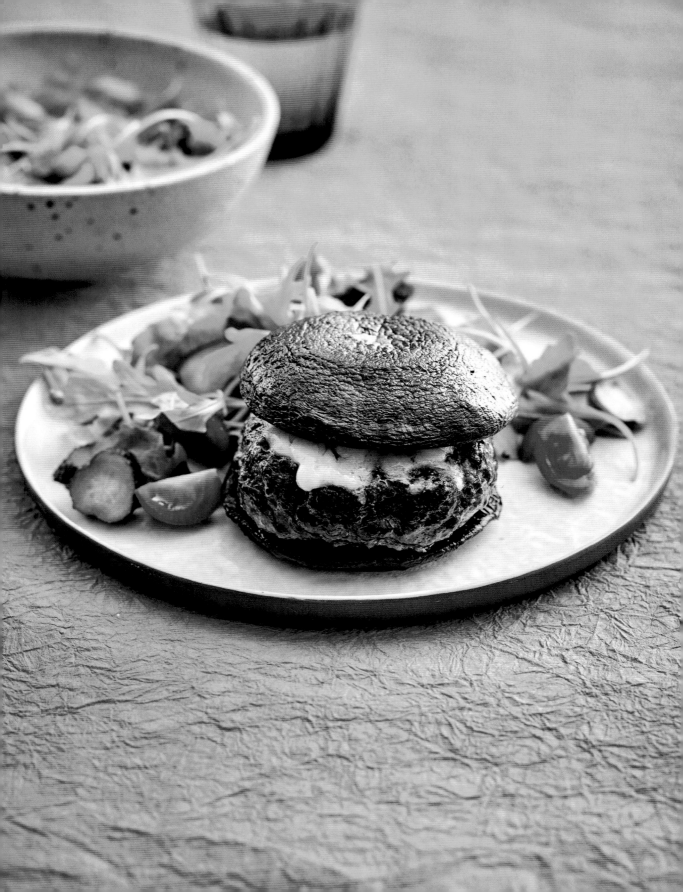

BEST BURGER EVER

SERVES 1

Ready in 20 mins

1 garlic clove
1 medium egg yolk
120g minced beef
1 tsp mustard (any kind)
salt and pepper
2 portobello mushrooms
1 splash olive oil
100g rocket
6 cherry tomatoes,
   quartered
4 cornichons, sliced
juice of ¼ lemon
1 slice of cheese (about 10g
   – it's got to be mature
   Cheddar)

I'm a burger snob, and proud. I used to waitress in Byron Burger so I've literally been there, eaten that. Here's what I learnt after eating about 300 burgers: a portobello makes the best bun; cheese is non-negotiable; mixing a little egg and mustard into your meat makes it so tasty.

Heat the grill.

Peel and grate your garlic, then stir the egg yolk and garlic into the minced beef with the mustard and salt and pepper. Use your hands to form a patty.

Pull the stalks off your mushrooms and turn them top-side down. Give them a dash of oil and some salt and pepper.

Slide the burger and mushrooms side by side under the grill. Both the burger and mushrooms take 10 minutes to grill, flipping everything over halfway through.

Plate up your salad ingredients. Dress the salad with the lemon juice.

In the last minute of cooking time, lay your cheese slice on top of your burger to melt.

Stack your burger in its portobello bun and serve with the salad.

SEARED TUNA STEAK

SERVES 1, PLUS
LEFTOVERS

Ready in 15 mins

1 drizzle olive oil
50g asparagus
   (about 6 spears)
50g kale
2 tuna steaks, about 150g
   each (one for now, one for
   tomorrow)
50g green beans
50g pak choi, separated
   into leaves
1 tbsp hoisin sauce

A tuna steak on a big bed of greens, a splash of hoisin to make it sing... perfection. Cook two steaks and reinvent one for tomorrow's lunchbox (see page 64).

Heat the griddle pan to high and drizzle with olive oil.

Break the woody ends off the asparagus and throw them away. Remove and throw away the stalks from your kale.

Put your tuna steaks in the hot pan and arrange all the green veg around them. Drizzle your hoisin over the veg.

Flip the tuna after 1–2 minutes. Keep an eye on the side of each tuna steak as it cooks. The sides should stay pink in the middle. If the sides of the steaks are completely brown, they will be well done inside too and not as juicy.

Plate up the green veg and top with a tuna steak. Leave the second steak to cool and then put in the fridge overnight. Tomorrow you'll love the tuna Niçoise on page 64.

CHICKEN AND CASHEW STIR-FRY

SERVES 1

Ready in 15 mins

1 onion
1 red pepper, deseeded
50g mushrooms
50g asparagus
    (about 6 spears)
1 tbsp sesame or vegetable
    oil
2 tbsp soy sauce (any kind)
1 skinless, boneless chicken
    breast (about 150g)
¼ cauliflower
juice of ½ lemon
salt and pepper
50g pak choi
1 tbsp unsalted cashew nuts

This is so colourful: stir-fried veggies and a side of cauliflower rice. And the next day the flavours get bigger and better, so double up the ingredients and you've got lunch tomorrow sorted.

Slice up the onion, red pepper and mushrooms.

Break the woody ends off the asparagus spears and throw them away.

Heat the oil in a pan over a high heat and add the onion to cook for 1–2 minutes.

Add the red pepper, asparagus and mushrooms to the pan along with the soy sauce and cook for another minute while you cut up your chicken into strips.

Toss in the chicken and stir-fry everything together for a few minutes.

Chop the cauliflower into chunks and blitz for 10 seconds in the blender – you're aiming for a rice-like consistency.

Put the cauliflower rice in a second pan, add the lemon juice, season well and warm through for 2 minutes (cook until just hot, then take off the heat to stop it going mushy).

Separate the pak choi leaves and add those to the chicken pan along with the cashew nuts to cook while you plate up the cauliflower rice.

Serve everything together.

THE VEGAN VERSION: Swap 150g chicken for Quorn 'chicken'.

COMFORT BOWL CHILLI

SERVES 2

Ready in 30 mins

1 tbsp olive oil
1 onion
4 garlic cloves
1 red chilli
2 carrots
2 courgettes
1 tsp ground cumin
1 tsp smoked paprika
2 tsp dried Italian herbs,
    or 1 tsp of each basil and
    oregano
2 tbsp tomato purée
100g mushrooms, roughly
    chopped
100g cherry tomatoes,
    quartered
1 tbsp balsamic vinegar
300g turkey mince
salt and pepper
½ cauliflower
juice of ½ lemon
1 handful fresh spinach
hot pepper sauce, to taste
1 dollop Greek yogurt
    (optional)

A big bowl of comforting chilli puts the fire back in your belly when you're tired. I choose turkey mince over beef as it's leaner. This recipe serves two; even if I'm cooking alone I'll make it in these quantities because I'm already looking forward to green chilli tacos (see page 71) or a burrito (see page 53) for my lunch tomorrow.

Heat the oil in a large pan over a low heat. Chop the onion and add it to the pan to soften.

Peel and slice the garlic, then slice the chilli (discarding the seeds if you like), the carrots and courgettes. Chunky courgette is fine, but cut your carrots a bit thinner or they'll take forever to cook.

Put the garlic and veg in the pan with the onion and stir your spices and herbs in too.

Cook for 5 minutes, then add the tomato purée, mushrooms, tomatoes, balsamic vinegar and turkey mince. Season well and leave to cook for another 10 minutes, or until the turkey is cooked and the tomatoes have broken down.

Roughly chop your cauliflower, then give it a quick blitz in the blender until it's the consistency of rice. Warm it through in a separate pan on the hob with the lemon juice and a pinch of salt.

To serve, plate up the chilli and cauli rice with a handful of fresh spinach, and throw in about as much hot pepper sauce as you can comfortably handle. You may like a dollop of Greek yogurt too, if you go too crazy with the hot pepper sauce!

THE VEGAN VERSION: Swap turkey mince for Quorn mince.

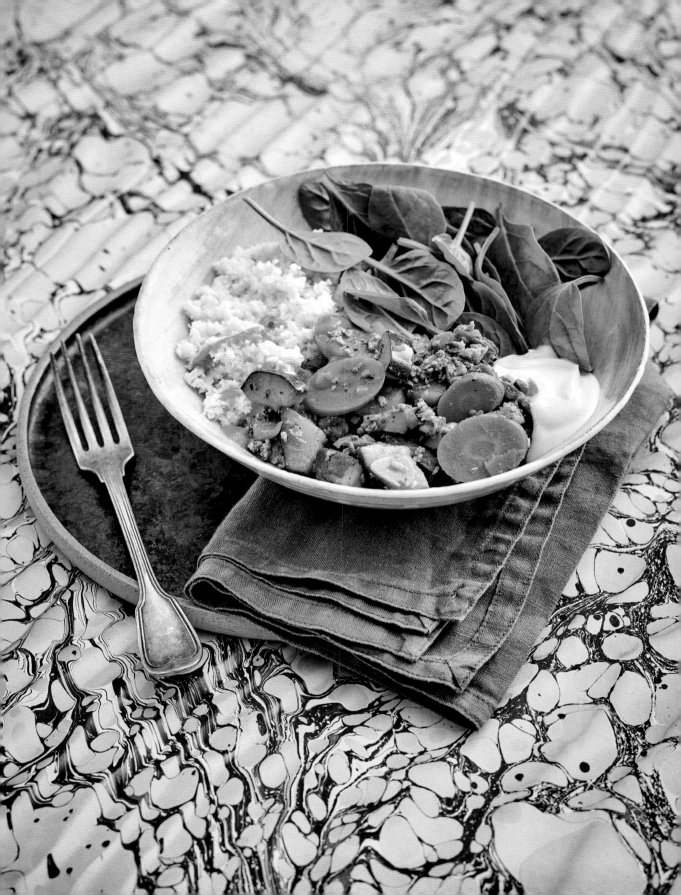

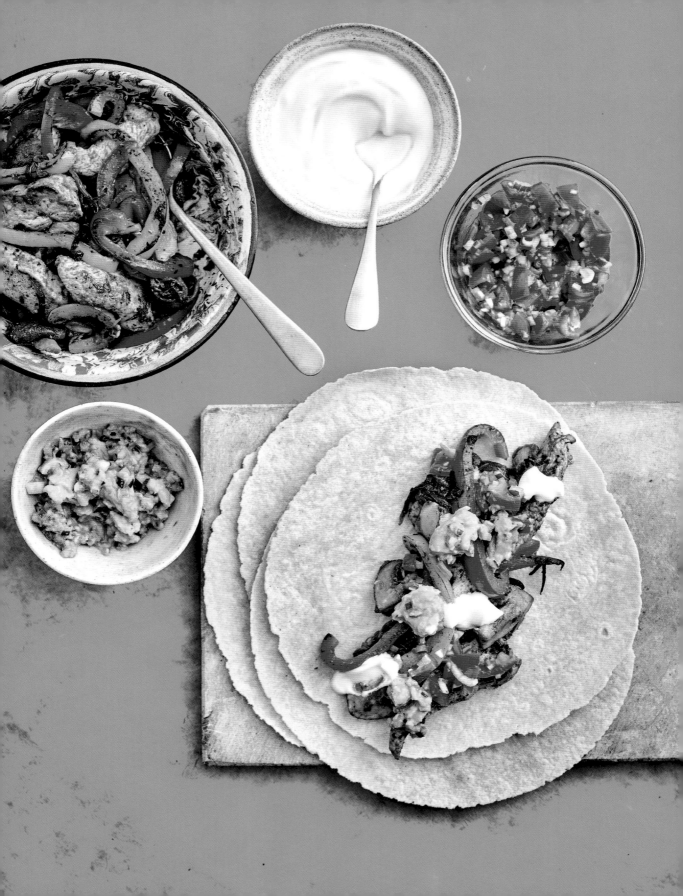

FAJITAS, REAL SLIM SALSA AND MY MAN'S GUACAMOLE

SERVES 2

Ready in 20 mins

1 tbsp olive oil
1 onion
3 garlic cloves
1 tsp ground cumin
½ tsp smoked paprika
2 skinless, boneless chicken
    breasts (about 300g)
1 red pepper, deseeded
1 yellow pepper, deseeded
100g mushrooms
salt and pepper
1 iceberg lettuce or 4 tortilla
    wraps

For the real slim salsa:
1 red chilli
6 cherry tomatoes
½ red onion
2 garlic cloves
1 dash hot pepper sauce

For my man's guacamole:
¼ red onion
½ avocado
juice of ½ lime

Instead of sour cream:
1 tbsp Greek yogurt

So easy and so healthy, fajitas are my go-to when friends come round for dinner, so I'll double or triple this recipe. I use iceberg lettuce as wraps instead of tortillas, but some friends are like, 'What? Lettuce? Shut up Gab, get the tortillas.' The joy of this dish is that you can make it work for everyone: you can pick and choose from the sauces too. Warning: I love my salsa crazy spicy.

Get your oil in a pan over a high heat.

Slice the onion and garlic. Add to the pan and soften for a minute before adding the spices.

Slice the chicken and peppers into strips and add to the pan. Halve the mushrooms, add them to the party and season well.

While they cook – about 10 minutes – make your dips. For the salsa, finely dice the chilli (removing the seeds if you don't want the extra heat), tomatoes, onion and garlic, then add as much hot pepper sauce as you can handle.

For the guac, dice the red onion and mash the avocado and combine with the lime juice and some salt and pepper.

When the chicken is cooked through and the peppers are soft, roll up into wraps with the dips and yogurt. I find it's best to do this at the kitchen counter before you sit down to eat. Otherwise, if loads of food is right there in front of you, it's surprisingly easy to eat more than your tummy is happy with!

SALMON QUINOA BOWL

SERVES 1

Ready in 15 mins

2 tsp butter
1 salmon fillet (about 150g)
2 garlic cloves
100g tenderstem broccoli
½ red pepper, deseeded
2 handfuls kale
1 tbsp frozen peas
1 tbsp cooked quinoa
salt and pepper
1 medium egg

'If you like it then you shoulda put an egg on it,' is my motto. I love this with quinoa which, thanks to the golden yolk, delivers like a protein-packed egg fried rice. Yum.

Melt the butter in a wide pan over a medium-high heat. When it's hot, add your salmon in, skin-side down, and cook for 4–5 minutes for a crispy skin.

Slice your garlic and add that to the pan.

Chop the broccoli into bite-sized pieces, dice the red pepper, remove and discard the stalks from the kale and chop the leaves as well. Add everything to the pan.

Boil a kettle for your egg.

Check the sides of the salmon; when the cooking line is about in the middle, flip it over and give it another 3 minutes on the heat.

Add the peas and quinoa to the pan to warm through, mixing with the vegetables. Season everything generously.

To poach your egg, fill a saucepan with about 5cm of boiling water, then lower the heat down to a simmer. Crack your egg into a cup (this helps it slip into the pan), then stir the water to create a whirlpool and slide the egg into the middle. Cook for 3–4 minutes, or until the white is set and the yolk is golden and runny. When the egg is cooked, use a slotted spoon to lift it out and drain off the excess water.

Stack the salmon fillet over the bed of quinoa and veggies, then place the egg on top. When the yolk breaks, that golden gorgeousness will run through your whole meal like the best sauce ever.

SIMPLE STEAK

SERVES 1

Ready in 15 mins

1 tsp butter
5 garlic cloves
50g mushrooms
1 steak (about 250–300g
  will give you enough for
  leftovers too, with 150g to
  eat now; sirloin is ideal)
salt and pepper
100g tenderstem broccoli
50g green beans

If you don't cook steak at home because you think of it as more of a going out thing, now's the time to change your mind. Why? Because steak is an excellent source of protein and, cooked right, tastes divine. Steaks are often massive, so feel free to reserve half of what you cook for lunch tomorrow – maybe a spicy steak wrap (see page 54) or a steak and fig salad (see page 75)?

Heat a frying pan over a high heat – you want it really hot. Melt the butter.

Peel the garlic (no need to slice the cloves) and quarter the mushrooms.

Season your steak.

Put the steak, garlic and mushrooms into the hot pan to start sizzling. Flip your steak when it is deep brown all over on the heat side – around 3 minutes for rare – and cook the other side for a further 3 minutes. (Alter the timings to cook your steak the way you like it: 3½ minutes each side for medium-rare and 4½ minutes each side for medium.)

Boil the kettle, then transfer the boiling water to another pan along with some salt and cook the tenderstem broccoli and green beans for about 5 minutes.

When the meat is cooked to your preferred pinkness, let it rest for 5 minutes. Your steak will reward your patience by being deliciously juicy and tender. Serve it with the veg.

CHEESY CHICKEN PARCEL

SERVES 1

Ready in 50 mins

1 skinless, boneless chicken
    breast (150g)
¼ red onion
½ red pepper, deseeded
½ courgette
1 garlic clove
40g Cheddar cheese
1 drizzle olive oil
salt and pepper
as much piri piri sauce as
    you can handle
1 tsp ground cumin
½ tsp dried chilli flakes
60g cooked quinoa

When you open this parcel, oh my word: cheesy chicken-y perfection. For lunch ready-made for tomorrow, double the quantities and pop an extra parcel in the oven.

Heat the oven to 200°C (or 180°C for a fan oven).

Loosely wrap your chicken breast in a big sheet of oiled foil, leaving enough space for the veg. Put it in the oven for a 5-minute head start while you chop all your vegetables and garlic and grate your cheese.

Take the chicken parcel out of the oven and open up the foil. Arrange all the veg and garlic in the foil around the chicken, sprinkle the cheese on top, drizzle with olive oil and season with salt and pepper and a dash of piri piri sauce. Close the parcel and bake for 45 minutes. There's that workout window you're looking for.

Just before you're about to eat, stir the cumin, chilli flakes and salt and pepper through your cooked quinoa and give it 1 minute in a pan over a medium heat to warm through.

Serve your chicken and cheesy veggies on top of the quinoa, drizzled with more piri piri sauce. Yum.

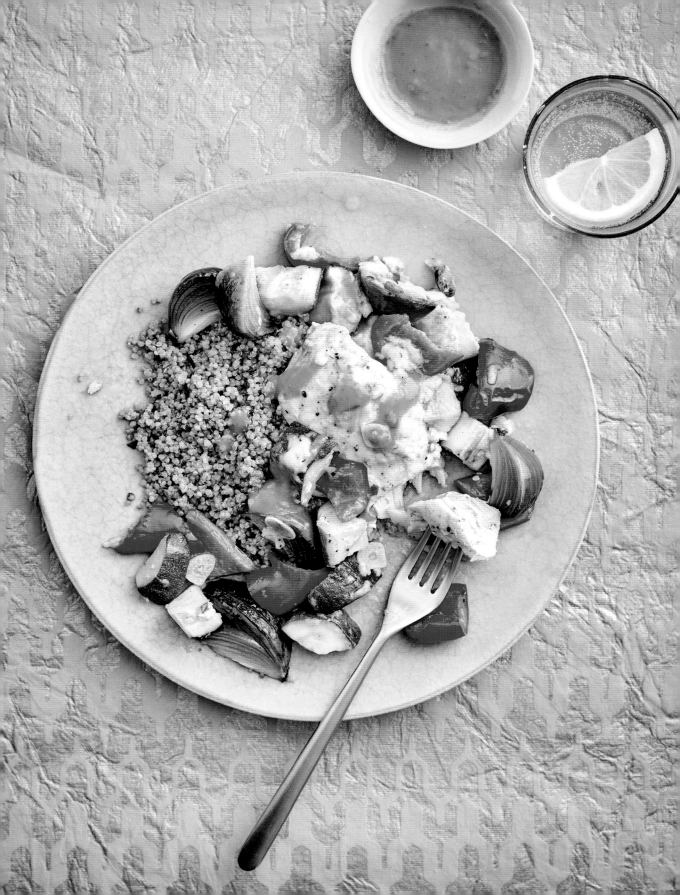

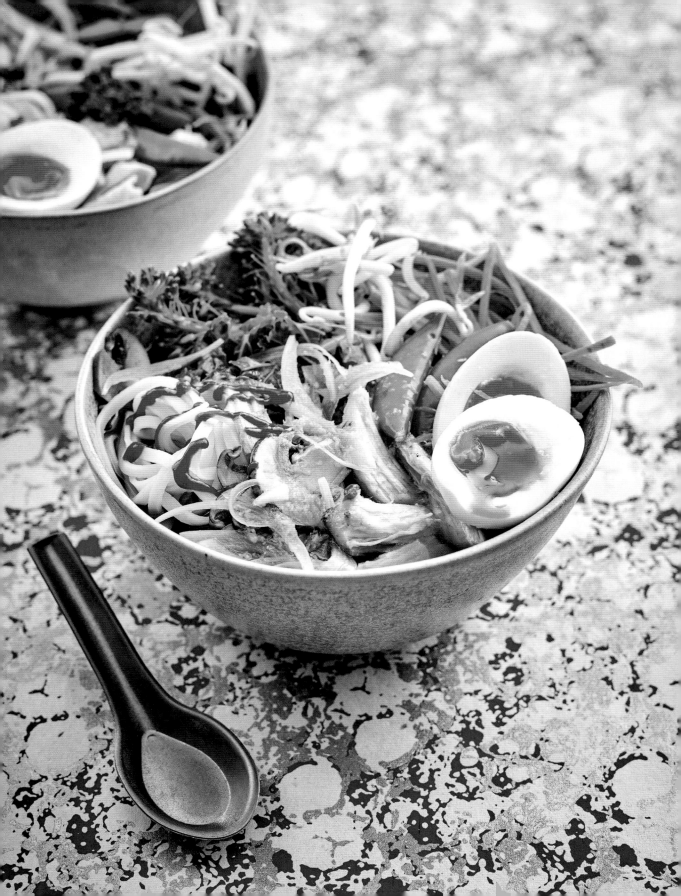

RA-RA CHICKEN

DINNERS

97

FOOD!

SERVES 2

Ready in 20 mins

2 medium eggs
500ml chicken stock
2 tbsp soy sauce (any kind)
1 onion
1 red chilli
4 garlic cloves
4cm-piece fresh ginger
100g tenderstem broccoli
60g sugarsnap peas
60g mushrooms
1 big handful kale
1 carrot
100g fresh rice noodles (if
    using dried/instant, follow
    the pack instructions on
    portion size and noodle
    prep as you won't need as
    many and you might need
    to soak them!)
2 cooked skinless, boneless
    chicken breasts, about
    300g, shredded
1 big handful beansprouts
hot pepper sauce, to taste

This is like a big hug in a bowl. If you prefer, you can swap out the rice noodles for courgetti. I don't have a spiraliser and cutting courgette ribbons is a bit of a faff, so I've gone for the easy option.

Boil the kettle and fill a pan with the water. Lower the eggs into the boiling water and cook for 7 minutes. Transfer to a bowl of cold water so the eggs stop cooking (sticky yolks are ramen's best friends).

While the eggs are boiling, grab a big saucepan for your chicken stock and soy sauce and pour them in.

Slice the onion and chilli, peel and grate the garlic and ginger, then bring to the boil in the stock and soy.

Add your broccoli and sugarsnaps.

Slice the mushrooms and add those too.

Simmer everything for 10 minutes.

Remove and discard the stalks from your kale and chop the leaves up into easy to eat pieces. Grate the carrot.

Add the kale, rice noodles, shredded chicken, grated carrot and beansprouts to the pan. Simmer for 3–4 minutes more.

Shell and halve the boiled eggs.

Divide the ra-ra chicken mixture and boiled egg halves between two bowls and drizzle with hot pepper sauce for an extra kick.

THE VEGAN VERSION: Swap chicken and eggs for 150g silken tofu (per person). Add 1 tbsp edamame beans per person for extra protein.

CHILLI BEEF STIR-FRY

SERVES 2

Ready in 15 mins

300g steak (sirloin is ideal)
2 garlic cloves
4cm-piece fresh ginger
1 red chilli
1 carrot
50g fresh pineapple or
    mango (if you only have
    canned fruit, make sure
    it's in fruit juice, never
    syrup, with no added
    sugar)
1 tbsp sesame or vegetable
    oil
2 tbsp soy sauce (any kind)
1 tsp honey
80g sugarsnap peas
100g tenderstem broccoli

Let me tell you, this spicy beef is not only beautiful hot from the wok, but it makes one punchy lunchbox for tomorrow. Trust me on the pineapple/mango thing: the natural sweetness balances out the spicy beef. It works. Trust.

Slice the beef into strips.

Peel and grate the garlic and ginger. Remove the seeds from the chilli, if you don't want your stir-fry toooo hot, and slice it up.

Grate the carrot. Peel, core and slice the pineapple or peel and slice the mango.

Heat the oil in a large frying pan over a high heat. Add the beef strips and sear all over.

Add the garlic, ginger and chilli and cook for 2 minutes.

Add the soy sauce, honey, sugarsnaps, tenderstem broccoli, carrot and fruit. Cook everything together, stirring, for about 5 minutes, then serve in a bowl.

This will be great eaten cold for lunch tomorrow too.

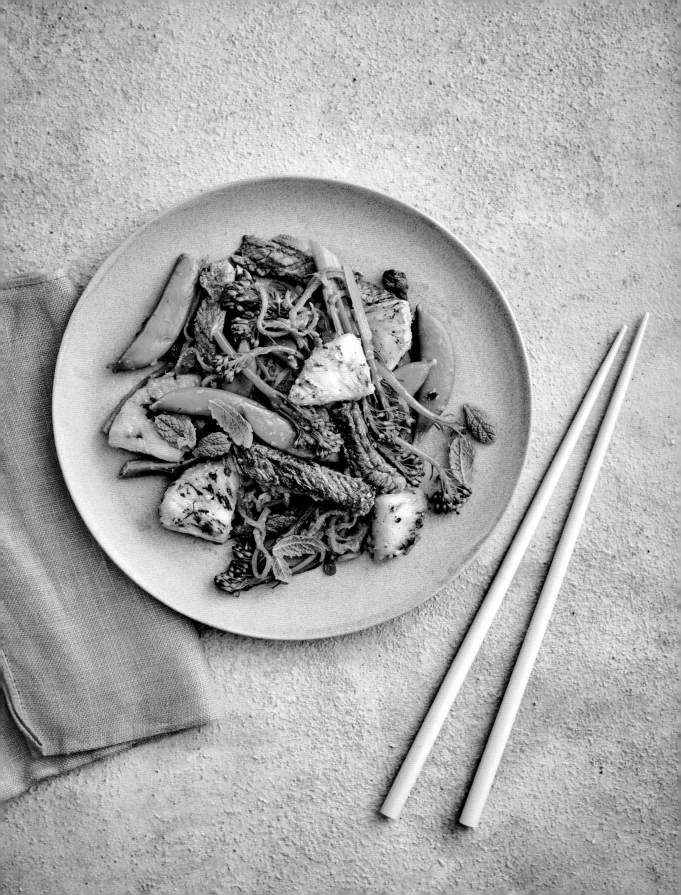

CHICKEN SATAY

SERVES 1

Ready in 15 mins

For the satay:
½ onion
2 garlic cloves
3cm-piece fresh ginger
1 tbsp unsweetened peanut
    butter
1 tbsp Greek yogurt
1 tbsp soy sauce (any kind),
    plus more if liked
2 tsp sesame or vegetable
    oil
1 skinless, boneless chicken
    breast (about 150g)

For the veggies:
50g kale
50g mushrooms
50g pak choi
½ red chilli (optional), to
    garnish

Peanut butter makes life delicious. Also, PB proves you don't need to be scared of fat: when you eat enough good fats your food not only tastes better but feels more satisfying. This is a great one to double up and have for lunch the next day too.

Chop the onion and peel and grate the garlic and ginger, then mix with the peanut butter, yogurt and soy sauce.

Heat two pans and add a teaspoon of oil to each.

Cut the chicken into bite-sized chunks – I find scissors easier than a knife. Coat the chicken in the satay mix and pour the whole lot into one pan. Stir-fry for 5 minutes.

Remove and discard the woody stalks from the kale and chop the leaves, halve the mushrooms and separate the pak choi leaves. Stir-fry for 4 minutes in the other pan, adding an extra splash of soy sauce if you fancy.

Plate up or, for visual effect (if you've got mates round), thread the chicken pieces on to a metal skewer, then pour over the rest of the satay. Arrange your stir-fried veg around. Garnish with the red chilli, if using, and then you're good to go.

EGG-FRIED CHICKEN

SERVES 1

Ready in 15 mins

1 tbsp sesame or vegetable
    oil
1 skinless, boneless chicken
    breast (about 150g)
2cm-piece fresh ginger
2 garlic cloves
2 tbsp soy sauce (any kind)
1 tbsp unsweetened peanut
    butter
1 tsp honey
1 tsp fish sauce
1 lime
½ carrot
½ red pepper, deseeded
50g sugarsnap peas
50g beansprouts
1 medium egg

I make this Thai-inspired stir-fry without noodles, because there's so much good stuff going on you don't need them.

Heat the oil in a wok or large frying pan over a high heat.

Cut the chicken into small strips and, when the oil is hot, drop it into the pan.

While the chicken is cooking, peel and grate the ginger and garlic. Mix together with the soy sauce, peanut butter, honey, fish sauce and the juice of ½ the lime (save the other half for wedges, to serve).

Give the chicken a stir in the pan. Then chop the carrot and pepper into matchsticks.

Add the sauce and all the veggies to the pan. Stir-fry everything for 5 minutes.

In the last minute of cooking time, beat the egg with a fork and mix into your stir-fry. When the egg is scrambled, you're done.

Serve with the lime wedges.

THE VEGAN VERSION: Swap chicken for Quorn 'chicken' and fish sauce for 1 pinch salt.

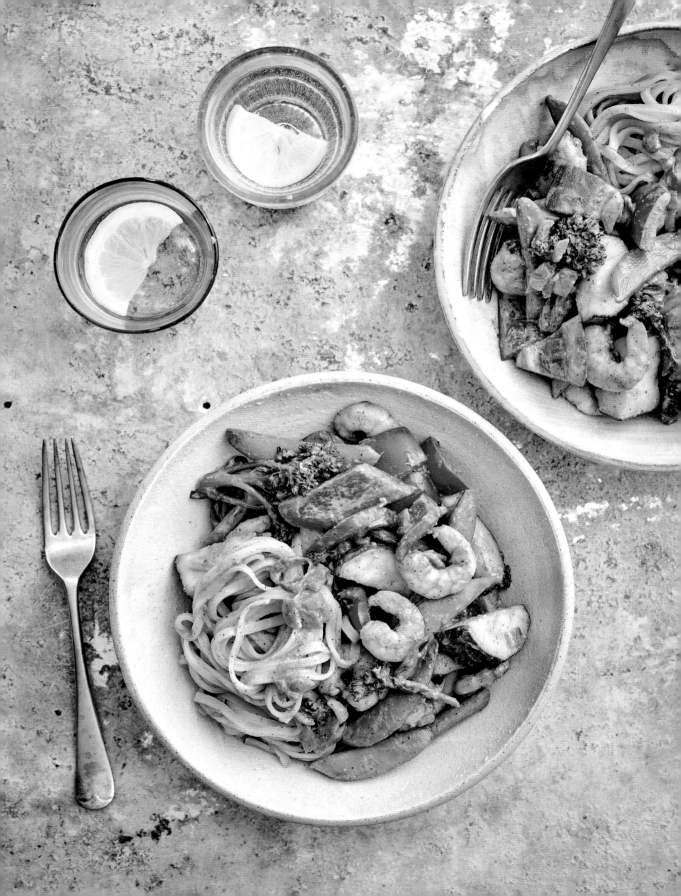

PEANUT PRAWN NOODLES

SERVES 2

Ready in 15 mins

1 splash sesame or olive oil
1 onion
1 red chilli
4 garlic cloves
4cm-piece fresh ginger
2 tbsp soy sauce (any kind)
1 tsp ground turmeric
1 red pepper, deseeded
80g tenderstem broccoli
1 courgette
80g sugarsnap peas
300g raw peeled king
    prawns
100g fresh rice noodles (if
    using dried/instant, follow
    the pack instructions on
    portion size and noodle
    prep as you won't need as
    many and you might need
    to soak them!)
2 tbsp unsweetened peanut
    butter

These noodles re-energise me after a workout and the peanut butter makes the dish taste properly decadent. If you've got leftover roast veg to use up, your noodles will be ready even quicker.

Heat the oil in a pan over a low heat. Then chop the onion and cook for 5 minutes. Chop and deseed the chilli, then peel and grate the garlic and ginger. Throw into the pan and soften for 2 minutes.

Add the soy sauce and turmeric, and stir.

Chop the veg into bite-sized chunks and chuck them all in. I love eating loads of colour.

Add your king prawns and cook for 2 minutes before stirring in the rice noodles too. Give them 2 more minutes, then stir in the peanut butter (it melts over the hot ingredients and coats everything, yum).

I could eat PB every day of the week; thank heck it's healthy!

THE VEGAN VERSION: Swap prawns for Quorn 'chicken' pieces.

PESTO-ROASTED COD WITH BACON

SERVES 1

Ready in 30 mins

1 cod fillet (about 150g)
butter or oil, to drizzle
1 tbsp pesto
juice of ¼ lemon
20g Cheddar cheese, grated
salt and pepper
1 tsp butter
2 portobello mushrooms
1 rasher turkey bacon
2 large handfuls mixed
   green leaves, like spinach,
   watercress and rocket

The day I discovered turkey bacon was a very happy one. It's lean but tasty. Bacon and cod are an awesome power couple. Throw meaty mushrooms into the mix and, yum, you're in heaven.

Heat the oven to 200°C (or 180°C for a fan oven).

Wrap the cod loosely in a foil parcel and place in a small ovenproof dish. Drizzle with a little butter or oil.

Top the fish with the pesto and lemon juice, then your grated cheese. Season well then carefully reclose the foil parcel (so you don't spill the juices).

Roast for 20 minutes, or until the cheese is golden and the fish is white through and just starting to flake.

When the fish is nearly ready, melt the butter in a pan, slice the mushrooms, cut the bacon into strips and cook them together in the pan until the bacon is crisp.

Serve the bacon and mushrooms with the salad leaves and the pesto cod.

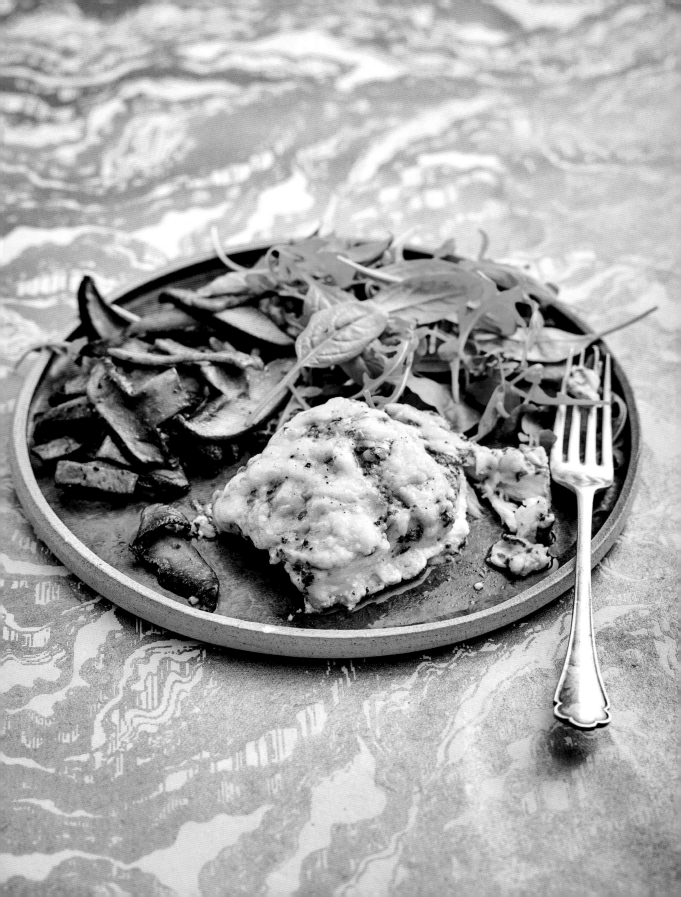

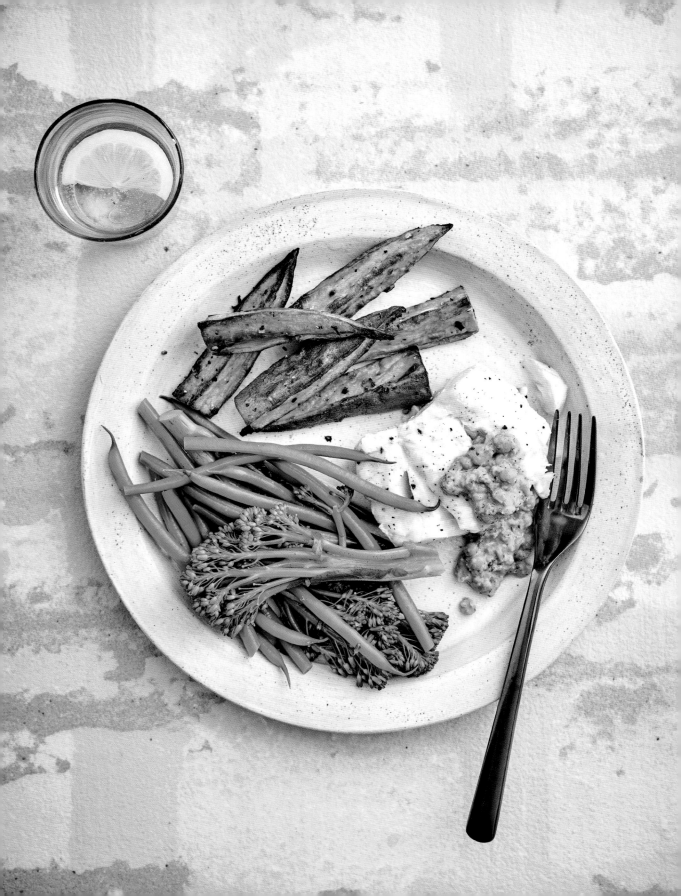

FISH, CHIPS AND PEAS

SERVES 1

Ready in 40 mins

½ sweet potato
olive oil, to drizzle
salt and pepper
¼ tsp dried chilli flakes
(optional)
1 skinless cod fillet (about
150g)
squeeze of lemon juice
50g green beans
50g tenderstem broccoli

For the mashy peas:
3 tbsp frozen peas
1 tsp mint sauce
zest and juice of ½ lemon

My family always used to get fish and chips on a Friday night. This is a decent healthier version without the fryer. It takes a bit longer than my usual recipes, but it is worth it. I'll just leave your fish and chips here for you...

Heat the oven to 200°C (or 180°C for a fan oven).

Peel and chop the sweet potato into wedges and lay on a baking tray. Give them a splash of olive oil and a good grind of salt and pepper, plus chilli flakes if you fancy more heat. Now get them in the oven to roast for 40 minutes.

In the last 20 minutes of the sweet potato cooking time, loosely wrap your cod in a foil parcel with a squeeze of lemon, a drizzle of olive oil and some salt and pepper.

Pop your parcel in the oven – the potato wedges will have shrunk down in the heat, so wiggle them over to make room in the roasting tray.

While the fish is cooking, cook the beans and broccoli in a pan of boiling salted water for 4–5 minutes.

In another pan boil the frozen peas for 2 minutes, then drain. Using a fork, crush the peas with the mint sauce and lemon zest and juice, a drop of olive oil and salt and pepper.

When your sweet potato chips are golden and your fish just beginning to do that beautiful flaky thing, serve with your mashy peas on the side. The weekend starts here.

CHILLI AND GARLIC PRAWNS

SERVES 1

Ready in 15 mins

2 garlic cloves
½ red chilli
1 big pinch fresh mint leaves
1 rounded tsp butter
150g raw peeled king
    prawns
salt and pepper
¼ medium avocado
100g rocket leaves
lemon wedge, to serve

Serve this with a fresh green salad or, if you're really hungry, add tenderstem broccoli and wholegrain rice. Typically I want to eat NOW so a speedy salad wins the day. The prawns taste delicious cold, so this is a good one to double up so you have some for lunch tomorrow too.

Peel and grate the garlic.

Chop your chilli (and remove the seeds if you don't want the extra heat).

Chop up the mint leaves.

Melt the butter in a pan over a medium heat and add the garlic, chilli and mint leaves.

Add the prawns to the pan and season well. Let them sizzle until they're pink all over; probably about 3 minutes.

While they are cooking, slice your avocado and arrange on a plate with your rocket. When the prawns are cooked, pour the whole lot over the salad – the garlic butter makes a delicious dressing.

Serve with a lemon wedge to squeeze over to really enhance all the flavours.

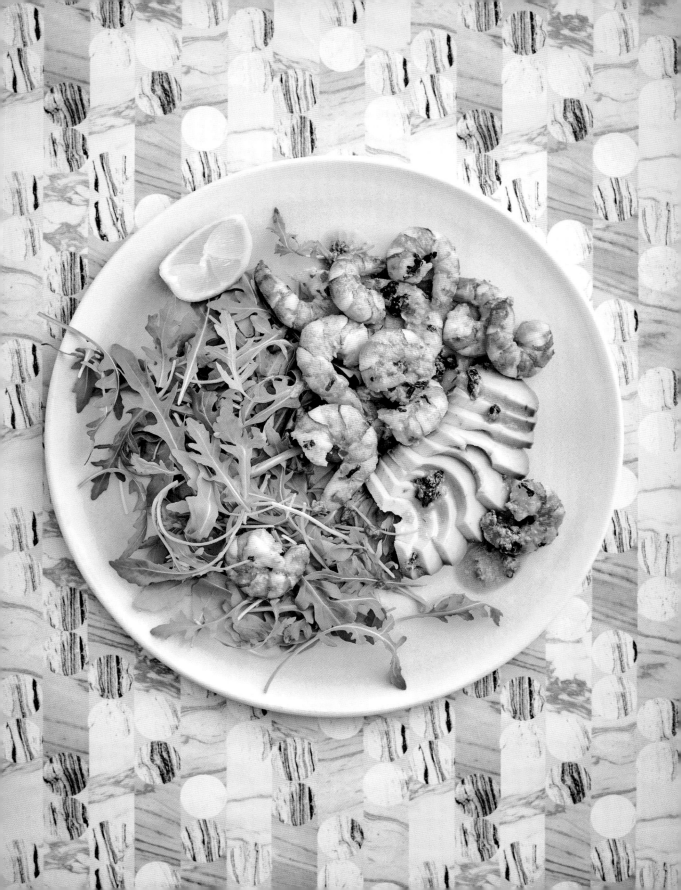

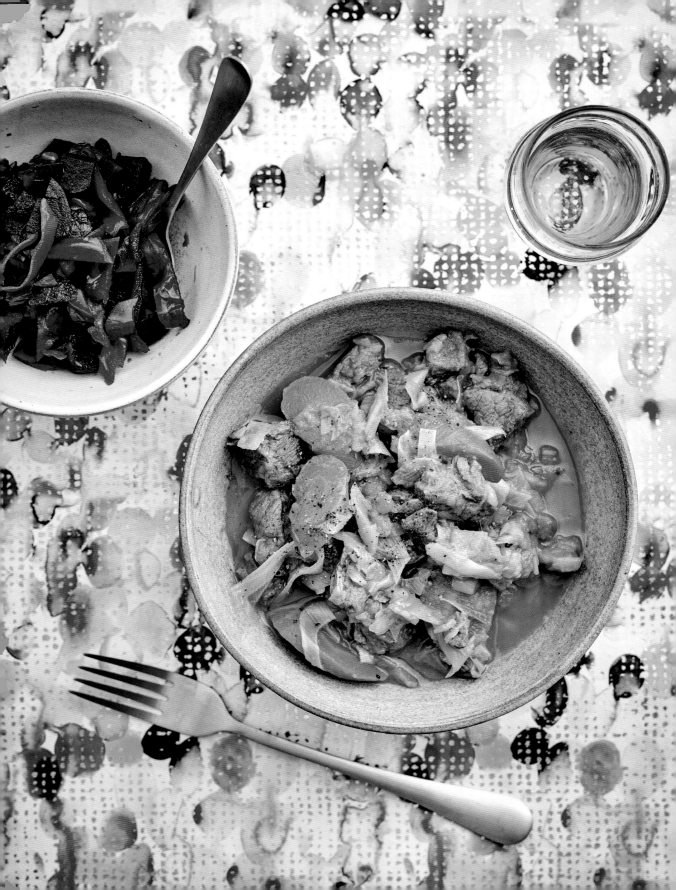

MY MUM'S SCOUSE

SERVES 2

Ready in 3 hours

300g lamb neck or beef
    stewing steak
1 tbsp butter
1 onion
2 leeks
2 carrots
1 sweet potato
salt and pepper
350ml beef stock
100g pickled red cabbage
1 cooked beetroot

As a Liverpudlian, I grew up on Scouse – a hotpot so good our city became famous for it. It's pure comfort food, and not just because it's the taste of home for me. Scouse is warming and hearty and full of goodness. This is an update on my mum's recipe with a few extra veggies, and skipping the bread and white potatoes. My mum swears by her slow cooker, but I make this on my hob. It only takes 10 minutes to prep, then you can leave it to cook over a low heat, come back and enjoy a lovely cosy dinner.

Cut the meat into bite-sized chunks, if you've not bought it already in pieces.

Melt the butter in a large casserole dish over a medium heat and brown the meat on all sides.

Dice your onion, slice your leeks and carrots, peel the sweet potato and chop it into 1cm cubes.

Add all the veg to the pot, season well and stir to mix with the meat, then cover with the stock.

Bring to the boil, then reduce the heat right down, cover and leave it to simmer for 2–3 hours until the meat is tender. Do you see a workout window?

To serve, add a side of pickled red cabbage mixed with chopped cooked beetroot.

HALLOUMI RATATOUILLE

SERVES 2

Ready in 1 hour

1 large aubergine
3 garlic cloves
1 red onion
1 courgette
1 stick celery
1 yellow pepper, deseeded
100g mushrooms
100g cherry tomatoes
1 drizzle olive oil
1 drizzle balsamic vinegar
1 tbsp tomato purée
2 tsp mixed dried Italian
    herbs, or 1 tsp each of
    oregano and basil
salt and pepper
150g halloumi
100g cooked quinoa

I love aubergines. This ones topped with colourful ratatouille and halloumi. Get this all prepped and in the oven, then have dinner after your workout.

Heat the oven to 180°C (or 160°C for a fan oven).

Halve the aubergine lengthways, then quarter it too so you've got four long pieces. Peel and halve your garlic cloves, then rub the cut sides of the garlic over the flesh of the aubergine pieces. Discard the garlic, or add to the tray of veggies for a more punchy flavour.

Cut the rest of your veggies into big chunks, except the cherry tomatoes which you can leave whole. Spread out in a large roasting tray.

Mix the oil, vinegar and tomato purée together, then use your hands to rub the mixture over the veg. Add a sprinkle of herbs and give it a good grind of salt and pepper.

Roast for 50 minutes – here's a workout window!

In the last 10 minutes of cooking time, slice the halloumi and griddle or pan-fry (no need for oil) until golden on both sides.

Warm the quinoa in a saucepan or in the microwave.

To serve, pierce your tomatoes with a fork and mash them into the mushrooms, courgette, celery, onion and yellow pepper to make a ratatouille.

Plate up the aubergine, spoon over the ratatouille and top with the halloumi.

The side of quinoa will soak up all the gorgeous juices.

THE VEGAN VERSION: Swap halloumi for 2 tbsp hummus.

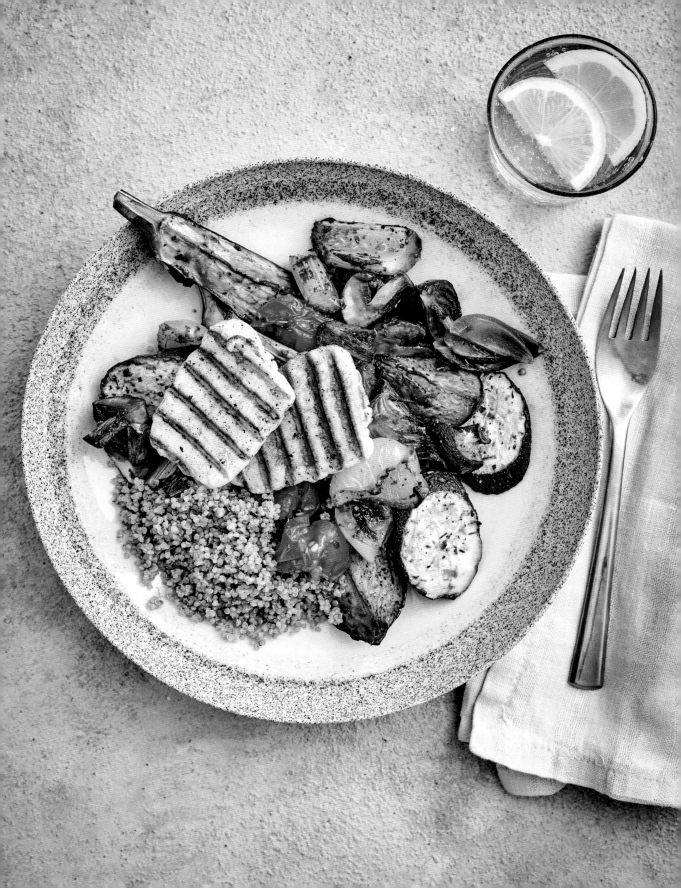

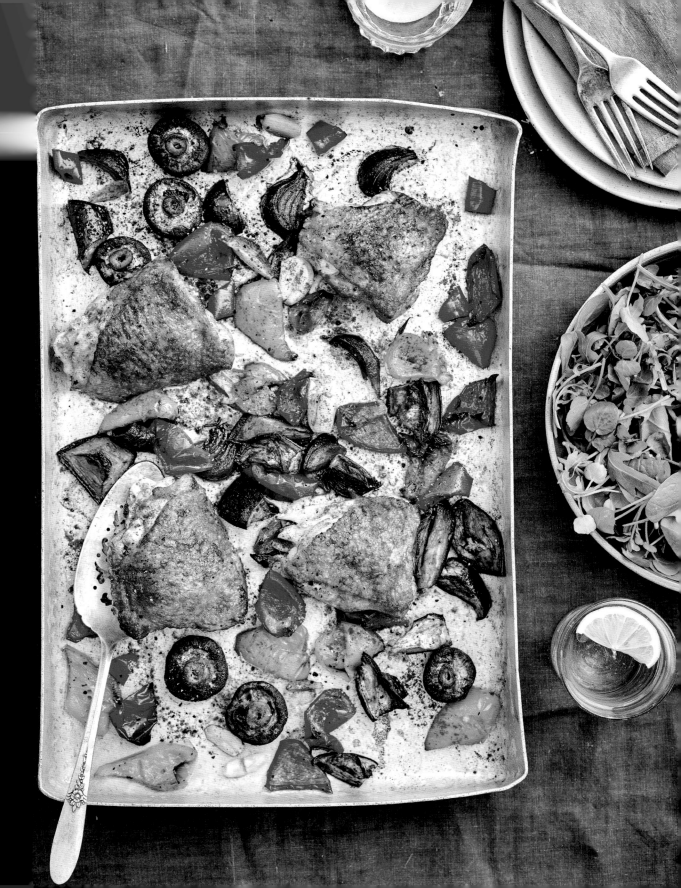

PAPRIKA CHICKEN TRAYBAKE

SERVES 2

Ready in 1 hour 15 mins

1 red onion
1 aubergine
1 red pepper, deseeded
1 yellow pepper, deseeded
1 red chilli (deseed if you
    don't like too much heat)
4 garlic cloves
100g mushrooms
4 chicken thighs (skin on and
    boneless)
1 splash olive oil
1 splash balsamic vinegar
½ tsp smoked paprika
salt and pepper
2 big handfuls mixed fresh
    spinach, watercress and
    rocket leaves

This easy-peasy traybake is my kind of cooking: fantastic ingredients you can quickly throw together to make something even better. It's so pretty: the full spectrum of sunset colours from yellow through to red and purple. I always make a double batch of this beauty as it travels well in a lunchbox.

Heat the oven to 180°C (or 160°C for a fan oven).

Cut the onion, aubergine, red and yellow peppers and chilli into chunks (I leave my mushrooms whole as they shrink down so much in the oven).

Peel your garlic cloves and press them with the side of a knife so they're slightly crushed.

Arrange all your veg in a roasting tray with the chicken thighs.

Splash with olive oil and balsamic vinegar, sprinkle with the paprika and season well. Stir the dish so everything gets a good coating.

Bake for 50–60 minutes – there's your workout window!

Serve each portion with a big handful of fresh green salad leaves. And a halo, because you're awesome.

SPICY SALMON

SERVES 1

This salmon is one of those great dinners that looks and tastes really impressive but is actually ridiculously easy. The longer you marinate your fish the better, so you could even take 5 minutes to mix the marinade in the morning, then leave the fish to marinate all day, ready to cook when you come home from work.

Ready in 1 hour 15 mins

For the marinade:
½ red chilli, chopped
2 garlic cloves, chopped
3cm-piece fresh ginger, peeled and grated
1 tbsp soy sauce (any kind), plus extra if needed
2 tsp honey

And the rest:
1 salmon fillet (about 150g)
1 tbsp vegetable or sesame oil
¼ red pepper, deseeded
50g mushrooms
100g tenderstem broccoli
50g beansprouts

Finely chop the chilli, removing the seeds if you don't want your salmon tooooo fiery. Peel, then finely grate the garlic and ginger, then mix with the soy sauce anad honey to make your marinade.

Spoon the mixture over the salmon in a dish, cover and leave in the fridge for at least 1 hour. Hello, workout window.

10 minutes before you want to eat, heat the oil in a pan over a medium heat.

Place the salmon, skin-side down, into the pan and add any extra marinade to the pan too. Cook for 3–4 minutes.

Slice the red pepper and mushrooms.

Flip the salmon over and add the tenderstem broccoli, red pepper, mushrooms and beansprouts to the salmon pan, adding an extra splash of soy sauce, to loosen the sauce, if you fancy. Cook everything together for 5 minutes. Serve.

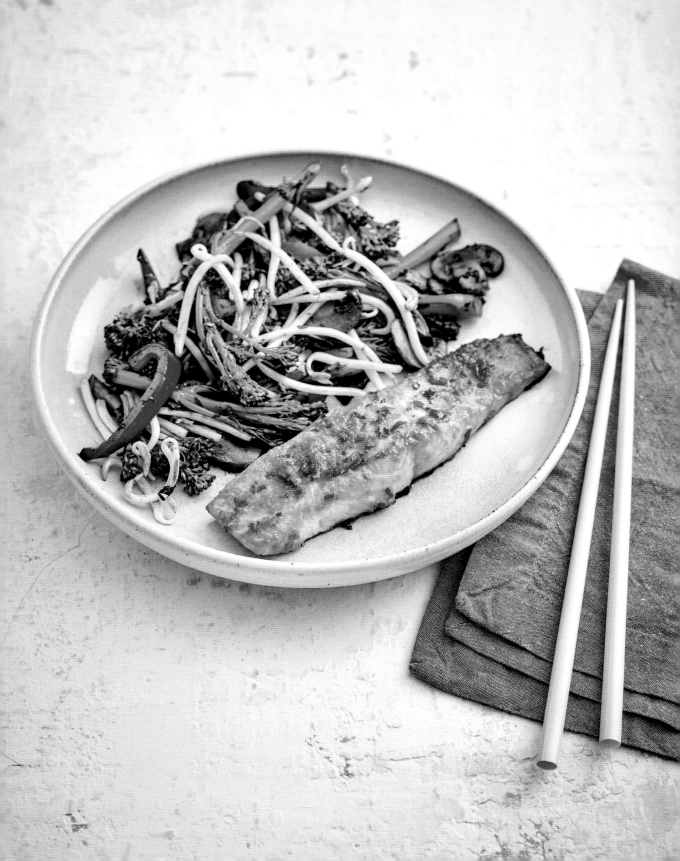

Snacks and sweet things

SHAPE UP YOUR SNACKS

Two snacks a day keep hunger at bay – Snacks and desserts are pretty much necessary for shaping up. Otherwise, you get so hungry, grab a doughnut and then what are we even doing here? So, feel free to enjoy one or two snacks a day on top of your three healthy meals. I love having a little something after dinner, so I always save a snack for then and think of it as dessert.

Portion control is key – I don't necessarily want a big sweet thing; just a little something. But I hate it when health experts advise you to eat one square of dark chocolate, like it's the easiest thing in the world. Because that square is physically attached to more squares, and the next minute I'm halfway through, and then I may as well just eat the whole bar. Gah! All my snacks and puds here are portion-controlled, yet properly satisfying so you won't feel the urge to scoff the lot.

Structure your snacks for success – In other words: be prepared. I know I'll be hungry every three or four hours, so I stash a snack in my bag so I'm not tempted to grab a packet of crisps or biscuits (or both) on my way home.

Snacks and desserts can be nutritious – I used to avoid snacks and desserts because in my mind they're automatically unhealthy. But actually, this is a way to get more nutrients into your body. I've included a fresh ingredient in all my recipes in this section so you get another of your 5-a-day in. You're welcome.

119

JAMMY PROTEIN BALLS

MAKES 12 BALLS,
OR 6 SERVINGS

These gorgeous raspberry-rolled protein balls are the perfect squidgy pick-me-up between meals.

Ready in 15 mins

100g unsalted cashew nuts
20g pumpkin seeds
3cm-piece fresh ginger
5 dates, pitted (I like Deglet Noor)
1 small ripe banana (or ½ if large), peeled
2 tbsp honey
1 tsp ground cinnamon
1 tiny pinch sea salt
2 heaped tbsp unsweetened peanut butter
50g oats
10g freeze-dried raspberries

Give the cashew nuts and pumpkin seeds a quick pulse in the blender – you want them roughly chopped, not dust. Set aside in a mixing bowl.

Now peel and roughly chop your ginger, slice your dates, then blend with the banana, honey, cinnamon and salt. There's no need to clean your blender – everything gets mixed together in the end anyway. Add the peanut butter, then give the blender an extra blast.

Spoon the mixture into your mixing bowl, then give yourself an arm workout as you stir it with the chopped cashew nuts and pumpkin seeds.

Chuck in your oats and give them a big stir too.

Using your hands, roll your mixture into golf-sized balls. Then roll them in freeze-dried raspberries to give them a pretty pink covering.

Line a dish with greaseproof paper and place the balls on it, making sure they don't touch. They'll firm up after 1 hour in the fridge, and last for up to 5 days refrigerated in an airtight container.

THE VEGAN VERSION: Swap 2 tbsp honey for 2 tbsp maple syrup.

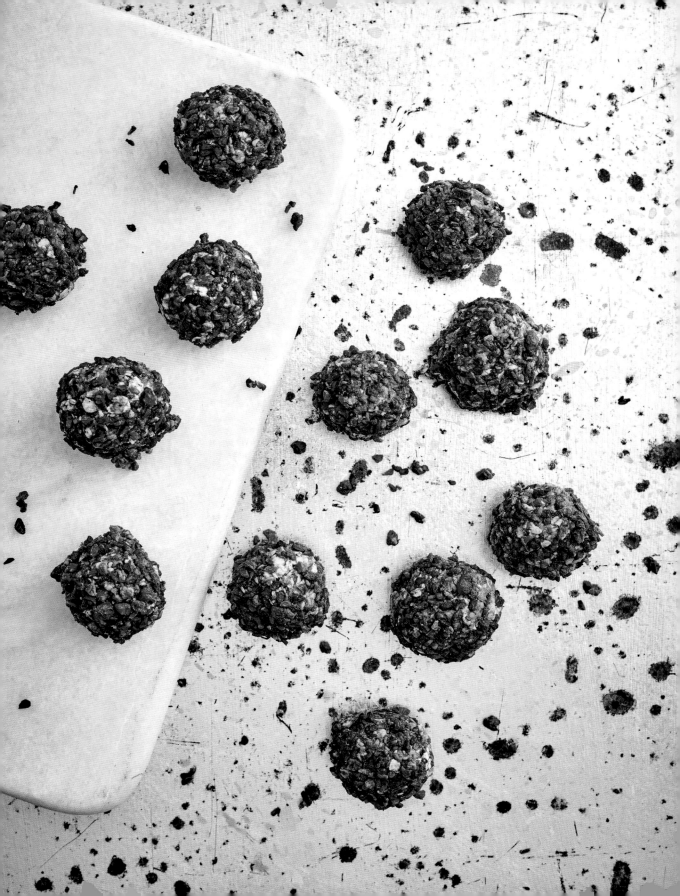

NATURE'S PROTEIN BALL

SERVES 1

Ready in 10 mins

1 egg
1 big handful spinach
dried chilli flakes (optional)

As you will have gathered by now, I love eggs. When you're making dinner at night, boil up a couple of eggs for snacks. I like my yolks sticky in the middle, with a bit of fresh spinach and some chilli flakes on top.

Boil a kettle, then transfer the water to a pan on the hob.

Drop your egg straight into the pan of boiling water. Set a timer for 7 minutes for a gooey yolk – I like it to be almost set, but still kinda sticky.

Scoop the egg out with a slotted spoon and put it into a bowl of cold water. This stops it cooking; otherwise you'll get a chalky yolk.

Either peel the shell off and eat straight away, or, leave it in its shell for protection and, when the egg is completely cooled, pack it into a small lunchbox. Add a protective big handful of spinach for padding and some chilli flakes for heat, if using, and you've got something tasty to munch on when snack o'clock strikes. I usually boil a few eggs together and store them in the fridge for the week ahead.

NO-COOK FLAPJACK

> MAKES 12

Ready in 15 mins

1 medium ripe banana,
    peeled
200g unsalted cashew nuts
    or almonds, or a mix of
    both
50g pumpkin seeds
100g oats
100g raisins or chopped
    dates
3 tbsp unsweetened peanut
    butter
3 tbsp honey
¼ tsp sea salt

A nice cuppa and a sticky flapjack anyone? These sweet'n'salt oaty bars can be wrapped in foil, stashed in your bag and whipped out when the 4pm slump strikes. Easy to make too – no baking required.

Line a baking dish with greaseproof paper. I use a 20 x 28cm dish for thinner bars, and more of them, but you might like yours deeper.

Blitz the banana with half the nuts and seeds in a blender, and roughly chop the rest. A nice little arm workout. Depending on the size of your banana, your mixture might need a bit more squidge. Try adding a tiny drop of water.

Stir all the ingredients together until they're combined, then use the back of your spoon to press the mixture down into the lined dish. You want it nice and firm.

Pop it into the freezer for an hour to set, then slice into squares. With some willpower, the flapjacks will last in the fridge in an airtight container for up to 5 days.

THE VEGAN VERSION: Swap 3 tbsp honey for 3 tbsp maple syrup.

RICE CAKES JUST GOT INTERESTING

SERVES 1

Ready in 5 mins

2 x large plain rice cakes

Topping idea 1:
1 tbsp unsweetened peanut
    butter
½ banana, peeled and sliced
1 tsp freeze-dried
    raspberries

Topping idea 2:
1 tbsp full-fat cream cheese
4 blackberries

Topping idea 3:
1 tbsp full-fat hummus
½ tbsp pomegranate seeds

Topping idea 4:
1 tbsp crumbled stilton
1 fresh fig, quartered

Honestly, if I'm hungry and someone offers me a dry, bland rice cake, I'll be like, 'Shove your rice cake up your arse'. But smother it in peanut butter, top it with blackberries, and then we're talking. You can swing sweet or savoury here, wherever your mood takes you.

Grab your rice cakes.

Load them up with so many awesome toppings that you forget you're eating rice cakes.

THE VEGAN VERSION: Swap cream cheese for oat cream cheese (yes, oat cream cheese is a thing); stilton for cashew butter, or garlic-flavoured cashew cream cheese.

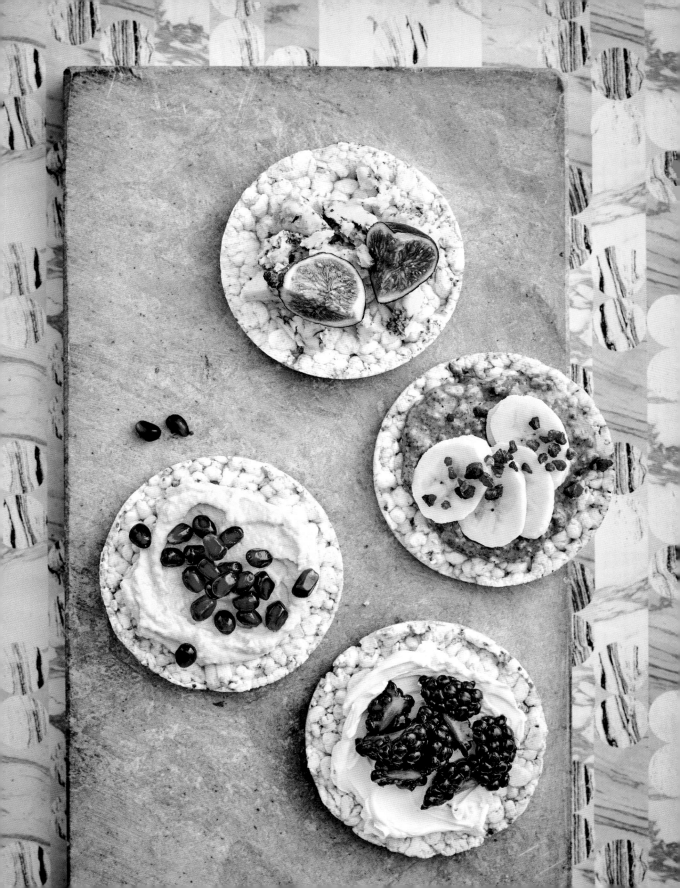

BLUEBERRY FRO-YO

SERVES 1

Ready in 5 mins

80g frozen blueberries
3 tbsp Greek yogurt
2 tsp honey
1 tsp ground cinnamon

You know when you've got period pains and all you want to do is snuggle on the sofa and eat ice cream? I reckon this 2-minute frozen yogurt is the healthiest possible way you can handle that. I love it that these are all ingredients I've got in my kitchen 365 days a year – there's no need to save this beauty for that time of the month.

Stir all the ingredients together until the frozen blueberries start to soften and make a purple swirl in the yogurt.

That's all.

THE VEGAN VERSION: Swap 3 tbsp Greek yogurt for 3 tbsp coconut yogurt; 2 tsp honey for 2 tsp maple syrup.

A BEAUTIFUL MESS

SERVES 1

Ready in 5 mins

100g strawberries
1 large rice cake
3 tbsp Greek yogurt

This is my take on Eton Mess. I swap out all the meringue for a rice cake, which gives the same satisfying crunch but with way less sugar. When strawberries are ripe, they're sweet enough. I also swap cream for Greek yogurt as it's higher in protein but naturally creamy.

Chop your strawberries.

Smash up your rice cake.

Swirl it all together with the yogurt. Eat and think of England.

THE VEGAN VERSION: Swap 3 tbsp Greek yogurt for 3 tbsp soya yogurt.

CLASS IN A GLASS

SERVES 1

This is good enough to serve when your mates come over for dinner. The trick is presentation. So simple.

Ready in 5 mins

3 ripe figs
2 tbsp Greek yogurt
1 small handful unsalted
    cashew nuts
1 tbsp honey
½ tsp ground cinnamon

Quarter your figs and arrange the first layer around the bottom of the glass, then use a teaspoon to dollop a little Greek yogurt into the centre space. Continue layering the figs and yogurt like this until the glass is nearly full.

Top with the cashew nuts, drizzle with the honey and finish with a sweet sprinkle of cinnamon. Tuck in.

THE VEGAN VERSION: Swap 2 tbsp Greek yogurt for 2 tbsp coconut yogurt; 1 tbsp honey for 1 tbsp maple syrup.

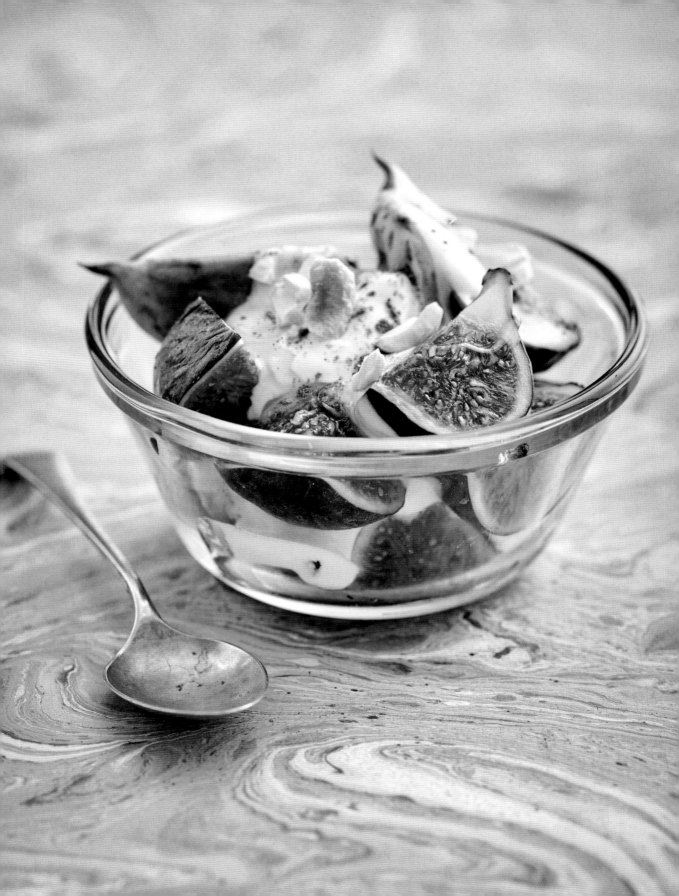

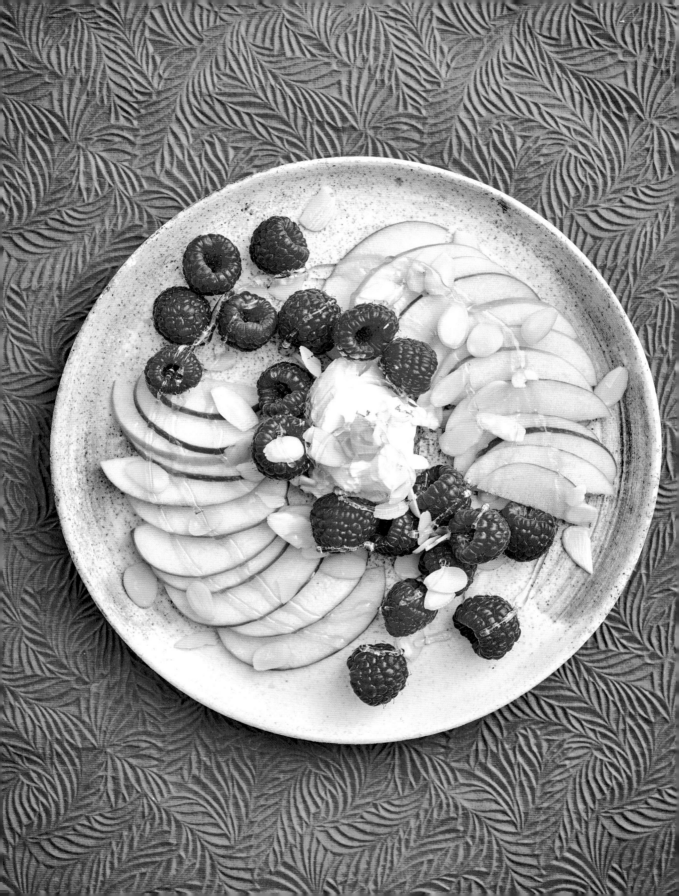

APPLE AND RASPBERRY PUDDING PLATE

SERVES 1

Ready in 5 mins

1 eating apple (I use Pink
    Lady)
80g fresh raspberries
2 tbsp full-fat cream cheese
1 tbsp flaked almonds
1 tbsp honey

I make this with Pink Lady apples because these apples have a cool name and, more importantly, they're naturally sweet.

Core, then slice the apple wafer thin and fan out the fruit on a small plate.

Scatter over the raspberries and dollop on the cream cheese. Sprinkle the flaked almonds on top and drizzle over the honey, then serve.

THE VEGAN VERSION: Swap 2 tbsp cream cheese for 2 tbsp soya yogurt; 1 tbsp honey for 1 tbsp maple syrup.

PURE PINA COLADA

SERVES 1

Ready in 10 mins

100g fresh pineapple or
mango (if you only have
canned fruit, make sure
it's in juice, never syrup,
with no added sugar)
1 heaped tsp full-fat cream
cheese
1 tsp honey
1 heaped tsp chopped
unsalted pistachios
1 heaped tsp pomegranate
seeds

I used to love this until I became allergic to pineapple.
Sigh. I've kept it in the book so you can enjoy it for
me; I'll make mine with mango instead. I haven't
spiked this with rum. But I won't judge. This gorgeous
dessert/snack hybrid is at its best when the pineapple
is most ripe.

Heat the grill. Peel, core and slice the pineapple or peel and
slice the mango.

Slide the slices under the hot grill, turning after 2 minutes.

Serve the hot fruit with the cold cream cheese, a drizzle
of honey and a generous sprinkle of pistachios and
pomegranate seeds.

THE VEGAN VERSION: Swap 1 tsp cream cheese for 1 tsp soya
yogurt; 1 tsp honey for 1 tsp maple syrup.

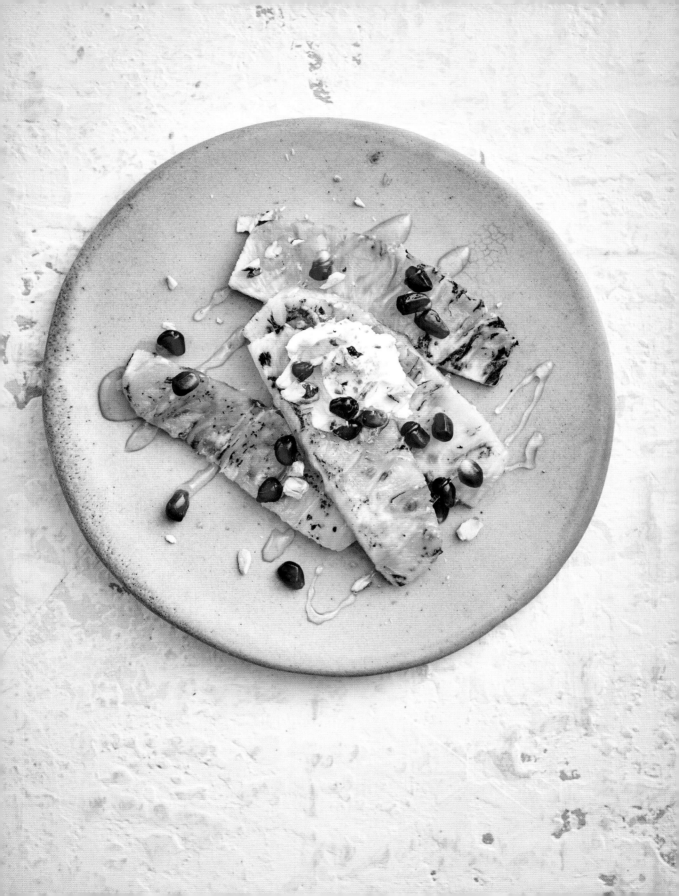

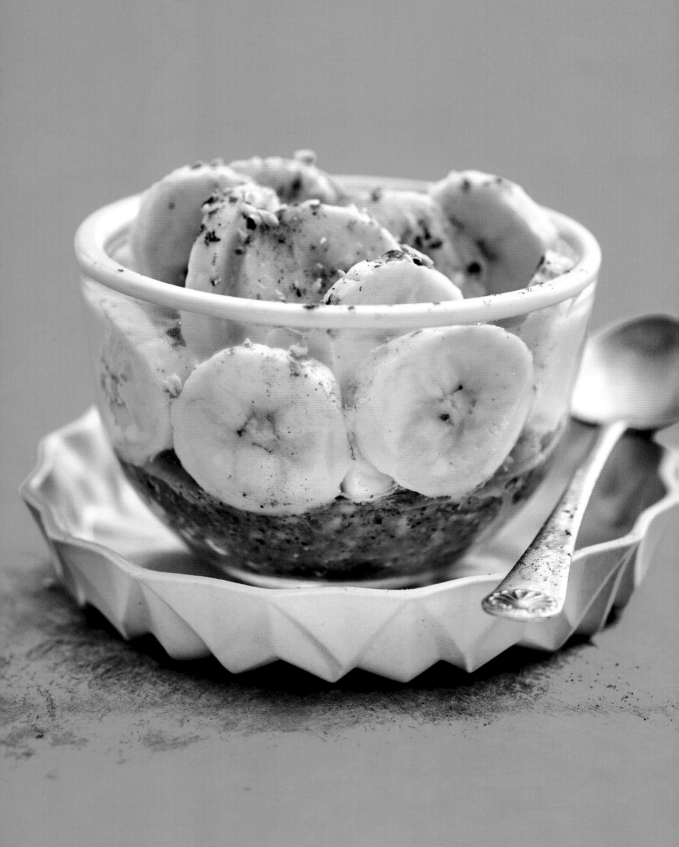

RAW BANOFFEE PIE

SERVES 1

Ready in 10 mins

20g unsalted pistachios, almonds or a mixture

20g unsweetened peanut butter

2 tsp honey

1 small banana, or ½ large banana, peeled

2 heaped tsp full-fat cream cheese

½ tsp ground cinnamon

This banoffee pie is full of healthy fats and natural sweetness, in just the right amounts to tell those cravings where to go. And it looks and tastes good enough to wow your mates with when they come over for dinner.

Roughly chop the nuts. Save a pinch for the top of your pie, then stir the remaining nuts together with the peanut butter and 1 teaspoon of your honey to make a sticky, crunchy base. Press into a ramekin dish with the back of a teaspoon.

Slice some of the banana to line the sides of the ramekin. Fill the space in the middle with the cream cheese, then slice the remaining banana on top.

Dust the top of the banana slices with the cinnamon, drizzle over the rest of the honey and scatter with the reserved chopped pistachios and/or almonds. Yum.

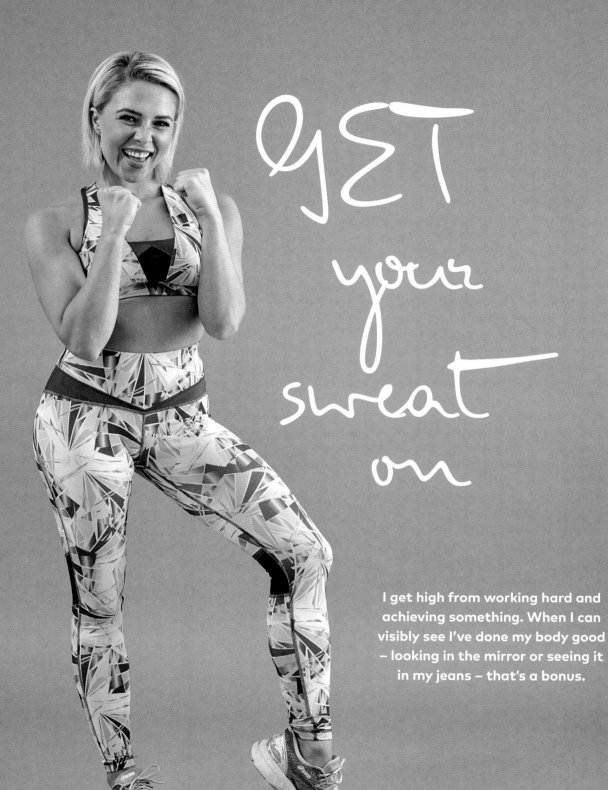

GET your sweat on

I get high from working hard and achieving something. When I can visibly see I've done my body good – looking in the mirror or seeing it in my jeans – that's a bonus.

Remember, in the time it takes you to procrastinate, you could have finished your workout already. Just start.

Sometimes, I can't be bothered to do anything. But I do want to shape up, so I'll have a word with myself: 'It's only 45 minutes, get your arse in gear.' I get my music on and get started.

I have to push through the first couple of minutes, then I start sweating and I'm like, OK, I can feel the endorphins now. Then my workout is literally done!

To keep you motivated, think about how good it feels to get your workouts done.

My routines aren't about looking pretty. They're about pushing you to your max. Working out can get quite animal! It's an amazing feeling to discover how much your body is capable of. And the end results? They're definitely pretty.

Feel proud of every step you take towards getting in shape. Stick at it, and you'll be proud of yourself every day.

Why these workouts HIIT the spot

- HIIT, or High Intensity Interval Training, is quick, efficient and easily done at home, in the gym or outside – and HIIT gets results.

- But physical results aren't enough: I want you to have a good time along the way. So I've got you a powerful mash-up of barre, boxing and 360° training to define, tone and sculpt your whole body from every angle, mixing in cardio for extra fat-burning.

- To keep things interesting, we'll combine high-energy moves like a really good exercise cocktail. I've created 20 workouts made out of combinations of moves, and no two combinations are the same.

- Don't worry: the moves are clear and easy to follow, and they're coming up in the next section. If you can work out in front of a mirror, you can check your form: it helps you get in tune with your body.

- HIIT involves exercising intensely for 45 seconds, then having a rest. I want you to work full out: keep going until you literally cannot do any more. I've included some variations in some exercises to protect your back, or to try if you find the main move impossible. Give everything your best as you'll only kick yourself for not working to your limit. I promise, you'll thank me later.

- In our workouts we use fast and slow moves to target your muscles in different ways. I call it 'tempo toning': fast moves like jumps and punches are fat-burning cardio, while slow moves like arabesques and squats build strength and muscle.

Look after yourself

- Do you have any injuries? Are you pregnant? Then please, talk to your GP before you try a new exercise routine.

- Before a workout, warm up (see page 143) and walk through the steps. This will help avoid injuries.

- Whatever shape you are in, always listen to your body. If an exercise hurts, stop. Take the pace down if need be. Listen to your body; it doesn't lie.

Your weekly workouts

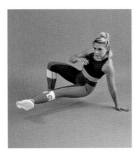

Each week you'll do five workouts:

1. **FULL BODY** – your 360° conditioning for overall weight loss and fitness. Focusing on reps, you'll use all the major muscle groups to build strength and burn fat.

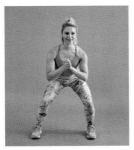

2. **BARRE** – especially good for core strength, this slow, controlled resistance training will sculpt your body, especially your abs. You'll notice the difference in your posture afterwards: holding yourself like a dancer can make you look a dress size smaller.

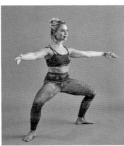

3. **BOXING** – my favourite, because boxing is my best stress-buster. I feel more powerful with every combination! The workouts are fierce, and really effective for cardio and over all body strength.

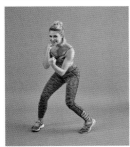

4. **LOWER BODY** – here's where we target-tone your butt and legs, the biggest muscles in your body. Extra bonus: firing up your biggest muscles means you rev up your metabolism!!

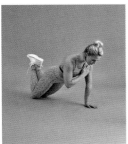

5. **UPPER BODY** – let's get those arms and backs sculpted and define those abs! To get the definition you want, repetition and control is so important in this section!

Your exercise questions answered

Q. I'm quite unfit. Can I customise the workouts for my fitness level?
Yes. Do the workouts at a slower pace to start with and check your form in the mirror. Safety is the most important thing. Once you've got your form nailed, speed up the combinations and up your reps.

Q. What do I do if I'm struggling with an exercise?
Look how many seconds you've got left on the timer – 45 seconds is not long in the grand scheme of things: you can do anything for 45 seconds.
   If you find an exercise really challenging, take it slow but don't stop completely. Remember, this is your body's way of saying 'You really need this.' That's when you get maximum benefits.

Q. What should I do if I forget what I'm doing?
If your feet get tangled up and you lose track of the steps, just keep moving for those 45 seconds. Jump up and down, run on the spot or shadow box.

Q. When is the best time to work out?
Any time is a good time. I like to get my workout in first thing in the morning, then it's out the way and it kickstarts your metabolism. Also, you'll probably eat better on those days: you've given your body some health, so you're thinking, 'I've already taken a big step in

the right direction, why would I mess it up with junk food?'
   Essentially though, it doesn't matter what time of day you do your workout, as long as you get it done.

Q. I'm busy. How can I magic up spare time to work out?
There's always an opportunity: first thing in the morning, in your lunch break, before you switch the TV on, when your dinner is cooking in the oven (I've factored workout time into lots of my recipes; you're welcome!). You make time to sleep, you make time for social media. So you can fit your workout in.
   Remember why you picked up this book: because you want to shape up.
   If time is really tight, then I want you to know it's better to do something than nothing. Do half a workout. You'll feel better. But best if you do a whole one.

Q. How quickly will I see results?
I think you'll start to see your shape start to tighten in the first week, you'll definitely notice a difference after two weeks and by the time you've completed the four-week plan, those changes will be like, WOW!
   Here's a cheeky secret: before a photoshoot, I'll always do one round of a workout. That blast immediately makes me look more toned – it increases blood flow to muscles and enhances them.

Q. What does 'go to your max' really mean?
It means pushing yourself to your absolute maximum. You'll get the best results in the shortest space of time if you give every workout 10 out of 10. It is intense. It's meant to be. Don't leave anything in the tank.

Q. I'm already pretty fit. Will these workouts really have an impact on me?
Yes. No matter how fit you are, you can always challenge yourself. If a combination is too easy, just speed up. I get really competitive against myself. If I did 14 reps last time, I want to do 15 today. Faster! Harder! Gimme an extra round! Push yourself.

Q. I love running/spinning/weight training. Can I keep that up?
I love all that too. A spin studio for me is basically Ibiza on a bike – party time! I've always loved running and deadlifts make me feel like a champ. Sometimes I'll dance so much on a night out it's a workout in itself.
   I've found that my workouts help me run faster, spin harder, lift bigger weights and dance until 3am still mad for more. What I'm saying is, give my workout plan a chance for four weeks, then incorporate whatever you were doing before and you'll feel even fitter. If you're already training, add this plan in and it will up your strength and endurance.

Q. What should I do on rest days?

I find active recovery is the best way to spend a rest day. If you're really hurting it helps to move. I'll do a warm up and my cool-down stretches, or go out for a walk. I promise you'll have fewer aches and pains, tightness and back trouble if you keep moving. The activity boosts blood flow and helps release lactic acid.

What else? Eat well, because you need protein to fix all the micro-tears in your muscles. And sleep: the magical answer to everything. You'll wake up tomorrow ready to smash another workout.

Q. I fell off the exercise wagon. Does it matter that I skipped a workout?

The world will not end. To get back on track, add in an extra workout on one of your rest days. And if you've accidentally skipped a whole week of workouts, pick up from where you left off and get back into your fitness routine. The occasional blip – however big – doesn't mean you have to give up. Get back on it.

Hit me up with any other questions at #shapeupwithgabbyallen

If you feel sore...

You may be experiencing DOMS, otherwise known as Delayed Onset Muscle Soreness. It's when lactic acid builds up.

Call me crazy, but I love that ache the morning after. It's satisfying: proof I've worked my body hard, and every muscle is responding. But I don't need to feel that soreness all the time, so here's how to relieve DOMS:

- Do active recovery as you rest between sets – walk around, shake your arms out.

- Breathe really deeply through the post-workout cool down as it helps you stretch out the soreness (see page 144).

- Tip a cup of Epsom salts in your bath. This relieves muscle tension and also helps you sleep well. You could splash out on fancy magnesium salts, but Epsom salts are cheaper and do the job.

- Treat yourself to a massage. Ideally I'd go for one every week – in my dreams. Realistically, you may have to ask a mate. Or use a foam roller to knead into those tight spots.

- Keep moving on your rest day. It's not a couch potato day! Any kind of movement releases lactic acid and makes you feel so much better.

IS IT DOMS OR AN INJURY?

DOMS can kick in from 12 to 48 hours after a workout. An injury feels painful immediately after training. If you're injured, please go see a physio or osteopath and get yourself looked after.

The 4-week workout plan

WARM UP

This dynamic warm up is a great way to get your body moving – yes, you have got time!

1. **SHOULDER ROLLS**: Roll your shoulders up to your ears then down into your back, squeezing your shoulder blades together. Do 8 big rolls forward; 8 big rolls back.

2. **ARM CIRCLES**: Stretch out to your fingertips, bend your knees as your arms stretch out wide. Do 8 rolls forward; 8 rolls back.

3. **NECK ROLL**: Belly button pulled towards your spine, knees soft. Keep your jaw relaxed. Roll your right ear towards your right shoulder and slowly take a big head roll around to the count of 4. Do 4 rolls right; 4 rolls left.

4. **SIDE STRETCH**: Stand with feet wider than hip-width, tummy pulled in. Slide your fingers down towards your knee, stretching the opposite arm up. Imagine your body is moving sideways between two panes of glass. Do 4 stretches right; 4 stretches left.

5. **HIGH KNEES**: Tummy pulled in, shoulders relaxed, jog on the spot. Lift your knees to hip height – do this 30 times.

6. **KICK BUTT**: Keep jogging on the spot, tummy pulled in. Flick your heels up to kick your butt 30 times.

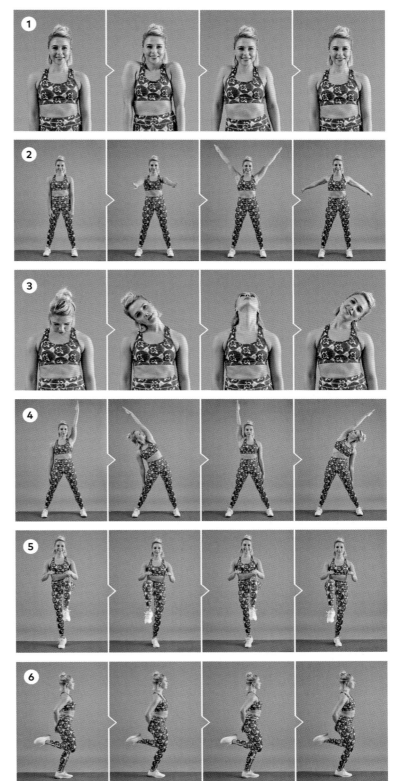

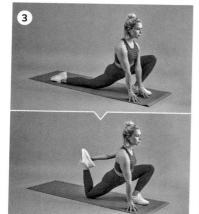

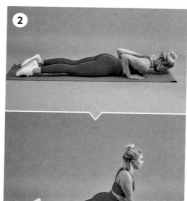

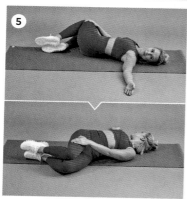

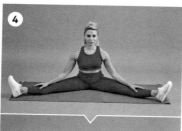

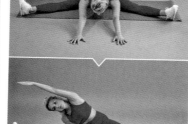

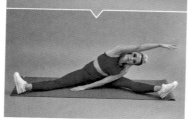

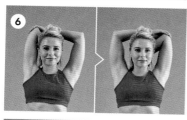

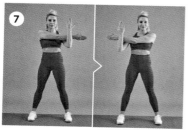

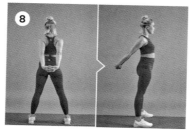

COOL DOWN

Give your body some love with these post-workout stretches. Hold each stretch for 5 deep inhales and exhales, then swap sides.

1. **BUTT STRETCH**: Keep your spine flat on the floor; cross one foot over the opposite knee; clasp hands behind your thigh and pull it in to stretch.

2. **AB STRETCH**: Start with elbows under shoulders; push down through your hands to lengthen through abdominals.

3. **THIGH STRETCH**: Lunge forward, lightly resting fingertips on the floor; for a deeper hip stretch, reach back and pick up your foot behind you.

4. **HAMSTRING STRETCH**: Stretch forwards between your toes. Relax your head and neck. Stretch over each leg; flex toes.

5. **BACK STRETCH**: Keeping shoulders on the floor, drop the knee to one side; turn your head to look in the opposite direction.

6. **TRICEP STRETCH**: Keeping shoulders down, bend each arm behind your head; gently pull the bent elbow with the opposite hand.

7. **SHOULDER STRETCH**: Reach each arm across your body; use the opposite arm to pull it towards your body to create the stretch.

8. **CHEST STRETCH**: Feet wider than hip width; clasping hands behind your back, push chest out.

WEEK 1

You're going to do 5 sessions x 45 minutes. That 45 minutes includes your warm up and cool down, so it's all wrapped up quickly.

HERE'S YOUR SCHEDULE:

Monday: **FULL BODY**

Tuesday: **BARRE**

Wednesday: **REST DAY**

Thursday: **BOXING**

Friday: **LOWER BODY**

Saturday: **REST DAY**

Sunday: **UPPER BODY**

Feel free to adapt this schedule. As long as you fit in five workouts and spread out your two rest days, you're winning.

Set up your timer

Use a HIIT rounds app to time your sets. I find Seconds easy to use (this isn't an #ad, just a helpful tip).

- In each workout this week, you'll do 5 different exercise combinations of 45 seconds each, with 15 seconds rest between each combination. That's one round.

- You've got a 60 second rest interval before you repeat the round.

- You'll complete 6 rounds in total.

- Add a halfway beep to your 45-second high intensity burst, if your timer allows it, so you know when to switch sides without watching the countdown clock .

FULL BODY

- Warm up (see page 143)
- 5 combinations, repeat each combination for 45 seconds, with 15 seconds rest, and 60 seconds rest after each round
- Complete 6 rounds
- Cool down (see page 144)

1. REVERSE LUNGE + POP JUMP TOUCH

– Step one leg back into lunge position, belly button pulled to spine, shin parallel to the floor. Return to standing; repeat with the other leg x 4
– Jump up, touch the floor x 1
– Repeat sequence

2. MOUNTAIN CLIMBERS + TOE TAPS

– Start in high plank position, belly button pulled to spine; straight line from head to heels; shoulders over wrists; pushing floor away to separate shoulders
– Bring alternate knees into chest x 4; keep hips in line with shoulders
– Reach for your toes with opposite arms x 4; keep back flat, lift hips to sky (bend knees and/or reach for knees if you need to)
– Repeat sequence

3. HIGH KNEES + SQUATS

– Run on the spot, lifting knees to hip height x 4
– Feet slightly wider than hip width, squat, keeping chest up and weight in heels x 1
– Repeat sequence

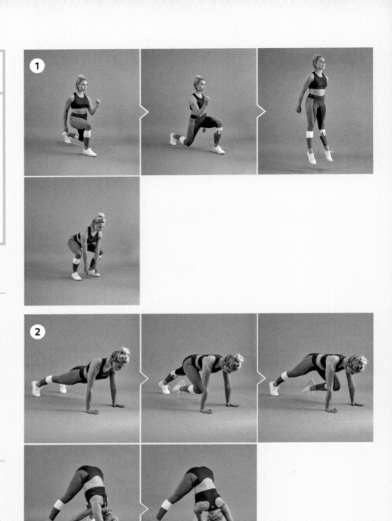

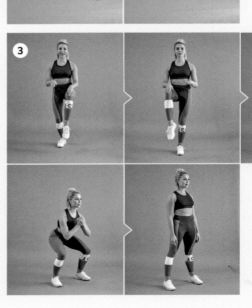

4. COMMANDO ELBOWS + PLANK HOLDS

- Start in high plank position, belly button pulled to spine; straight line from head to heels; shoulders over wrists; pushing floor away to separate shoulders for 4 counts
- Come down on to elbows, one arm at a time into elbow plank
- Push up from elbows to palms returning to high plank
- Hold plank for 4 counts
- Repeat sequence

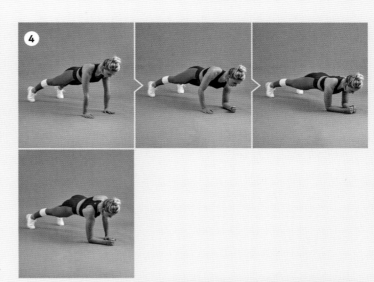

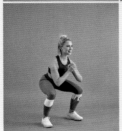

5. IN + OUT SQUATS

- From standing, feet hip width apart, squat, keeping your chest up and weight in heels x 1
- Jump feet to a narrow squat x 1 Jump back out, squat. Go lower!
- Repeat sequence

[Rest for 60 seconds before repeating the full body circuit.]

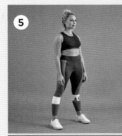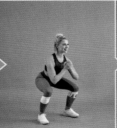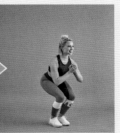

Completed 6 rounds? Boom! Now cool down with your post-workout stretches (see page 144)

>>>>>>

BARRE

- Warm up (see page 143)
- 5 combinations, with 15 seconds rest between each combination and 60 seconds rest after each round
- Complete 6 rounds
- Cool down (see page 144)

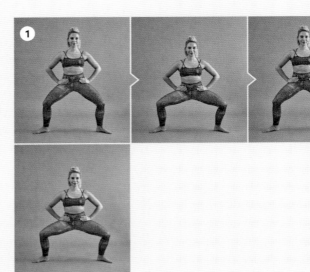

1. PLIÉ + PULSE

- Start in second position; feet turned out (at 10 to 2); belly button pulled to spine; shoulders down
- Drop butt down to plié keeping your spine straight; tail bone pointing to the floor (don't arch your back) x 4
- Hold the last plié and pulse x 4; tiny movements but you'll feel the burn
- Repeat sequence

2. PLIÉ JUMPS + PULSE ARMS

- This time, jump your plié, landing with bent knees and spine straight x 4
- Hold last plié down as deep as you can go without arching your back; pulse arms up x 4
- Repeat sequence

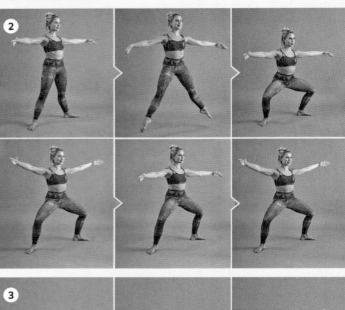

3. SLOW TRICEP PRESS + HOLD

- Start in high plank position, resting on knees; belly button pulled to spine; straight line from head to knees; shoulders over wrists; pushing the floor away to separate the shoulder blades
- Bend arms to press, s-l-o-w-l-y, keeping elbows tucked in (as low as you can) x 4
- On 4th press, hold for 4 counts
- Repeat sequence

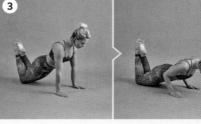
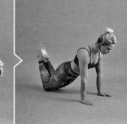

4. CRUNCHES + BICYCLE LEGS

- Start in table top, belly button pulled to spine, hands behind ears, head and shoulders lifted to crunch. Hold position
- Move one elbow to opposite knee, extending the other leg away (not knee to elbow) x 4
- Swap legs, holding crunch
- Repeat sequence

5. ARABESQUE + LEG LIFTS

- From standing, with legs slightly bent (don't lock knees), belly button pulled to spine, use your glute and hamstring to raise one leg up for the count of 4 and lower for the count of 4
- Try not to rest toe on the floor between lifts, or lean on the chair
- Switch to the other leg at halfway time

[Rest for 60 seconds before repeating the barre circuit. It's only 6 rounds; you can do it.]

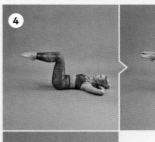
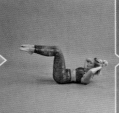
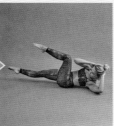
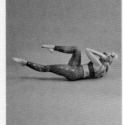
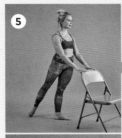
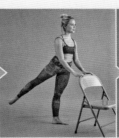
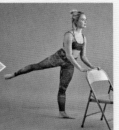
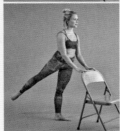

Now you've done the full 6 rounds, luxuriate in your post-workout cool down stretches...
(see page 144)
>>>>>>

BOXING

- Warm up (see page 143)
- 5 combinations, with 15 seconds rest between each combination and 60 seconds rest after each round
- Complete 6 rounds
- Cool down (see page 144)

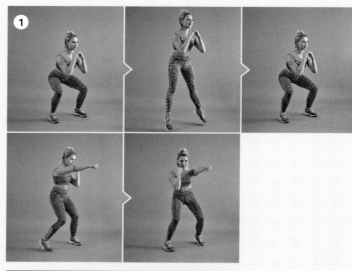

1. SQUAT JUMP + JAB

– From a wide stance, lower into a squat, keeping your chest lifted, weight in heels and your boxing guard up
– Perform x 4 strong jabs, staying in your squat
– Push through your feet to squat jump
– Land back into squat
– Repeat sequence

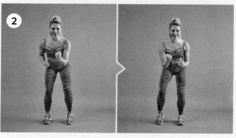

2. FAST FEET + UPPER CUTS

– Light on your toes, run on the spot as quick as you can (towards the bar for last orders – ha!)
– Punch from underneath as you run. Put some welly into it! Keep going

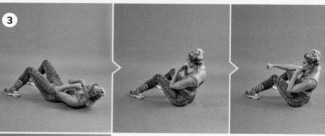

3. HALF CRUNCH + JAB CROSS

– Sit up halfway, pulling belly button into spine
– Twisting your torso, jab arms over opposite knees x 2
– Lower back to floor
– Repeat sequence

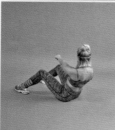

4. FAKE SKIPPING HIGH + LOW

- No rope required. Squeeze elbows in to your sides; stay light on your toes; relax shoulders
- Perform 4 high jumps, really pick your feet up; bend your knees on landing
- Now 4 low jumps, fast
- Repeat sequence

5. PLANK + UPPER CUTS

- Start in high plank position, belly button pulled to spine; straight line from head to heels; shoulders over wrists; pushing floor away to separate shoulders
- Hold for 4 counts
- Punch underneath with each arm x 4 (do this on your knees if you need to). Nothing moves apart from your arms
- Repeat sequence

[Rest for 60 seconds before repeating the boxing circuit. You've got 6 rounds in total.]

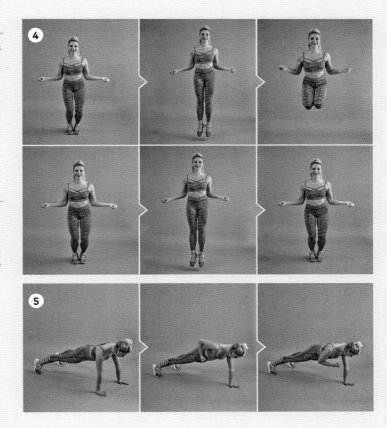

Smashed 6 rounds? Amazing! Now cool down with your post-workout stretches...
(see page 144)
>>>>>>

151

WEEK 1

LOWER BODY

- Warm up (see page 143)
- 5 combinations, with 15 seconds rest between each combination and 60 seconds rest after each round
- Complete 6 rounds
- Cool down (see page 144)

1. SQUAT + PULSES

– From a wide stance, lower into a squat keeping your chest up, weight in heels
– Hold the squat and pulse x 4; squeeze your butt to stand
– Repeat sequence

2. POWER KNEE LUNGES + REACH

– Step one leg back into lunge position, belly button pulled to spine, shin parallel to the floor; arms reaching overhead
– Drive the back leg up to your chest, pulling your hands down. Imagine smashing a brick between your hands
– Repeat until halfway time then switch legs

3. BUTT BRIDGE + PULSE

– Lying on floor, feet hip width apart, heels down, squeezing your butt, pulling belly button into spine, lift your hips to the sky
– Lower your butt to hover an inch off the floor
– Squeeze back up to the sky. Do this 4 times
– Hold the last one up and pulse up x 4
– Repeat sequence

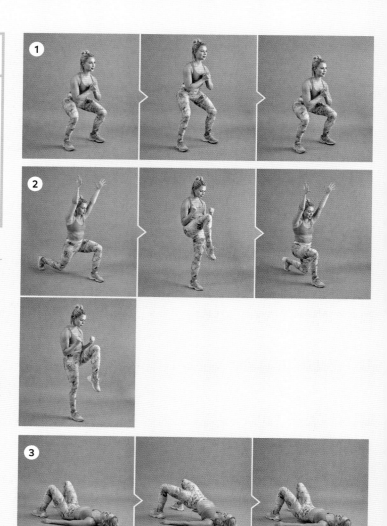
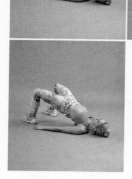

4. LONG JUMP + FAST FEET

– Jump forward, as far as you can.
Land in squat position, chest up,
weight in heels
– As quick as you can, staying in low
squat position, run back to the
start position
– Repeat sequence

5. LEG EXTENSION + PULSE

– On all fours, back flat, belly
button pulled into spine, shoulders
away from ears, extend one leg
behind you x 4
– Hold last one out and pulse your
heel to the sky x 4
– Repeat sequence until halfway
time then swap legs

[Rest for 60 seconds before
repeating the lower body circuit.
You've got 6 rounds in total.]

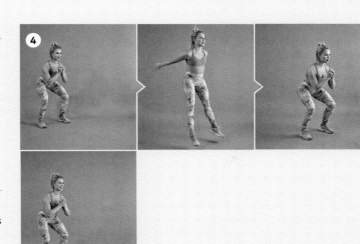

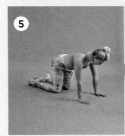
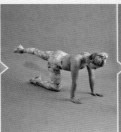
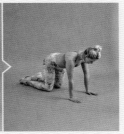

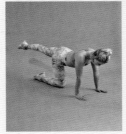

**Completed 6 rounds?
Awesome! Now cool
down with your post-
workout stretches (see
page 144)**

>>>>>>

UPPER BODY

- Warm up (see page 143)
- 5 combinations, with 15 seconds rest between each combination and 60 seconds rest after each round
- Complete 6 rounds
- Cool down (see page 144)

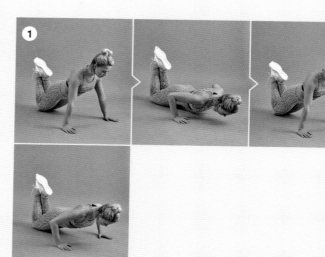

1. PRESS ON KNEES + HOLD

- Start in high plank position, with your hands wider than your shoulders, straight line from top of head to knees
- Lower chest down towards floor as far as you can go, press through your hands to start position x 4
- Press again and hold as low as you can for 4 counts, then push back up. Repeat sequence

2. HUNDREDS + SIDE REACHES

- Lying on floor, feet hip width apart, heels down, squeezing your butt, pulling belly button into spine, lift shoulders off floor and relax your neck
- With fingers reaching to heels, pulse your hands down x 4
- Then reach for alternate ankles x 4, squeezing ribs to hips
- Repeat sequence

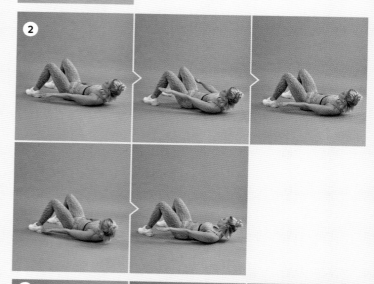

3. SUPERGIRL + TOUCH

- On all fours, back flat, belly button pulled into spine, shoulders away from ears
- With control, stretch one arm and opposite leg in line with your torso
- Squeeze your abs bringing your elbow to touch opposite knee. Extend back out; repeat until halfway time then swap sides!

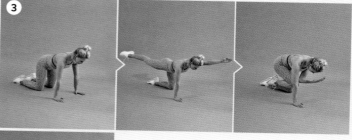

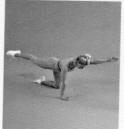

4. PLANK SHOULDER TAP + HOLD

- Start in high plank position, resting on knees
- Tap hand to opposite shoulder x 4
- Hold in plank for a count of 4
- Repeat, holding core strong throughout
- If you want to challenge yourself further, try in high plank

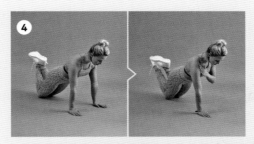

5. SLOW TRICEP DIPS + FAST RAISE

- Weight equally in hands and heels, fingers pointing forward or sideways, shoulders away from ears, elbows tucked in, bend arms to lower your butt s-l-o-w-l-y for a count of 4
- Make sure your elbows stay pointed behind you. Push up fast without locking your elbows
- Repeat and feel the burn...

[Rest for 60 seconds before repeating the upper body circuit.]

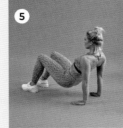
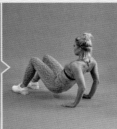
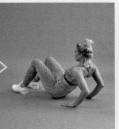
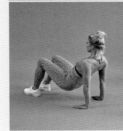

6 rounds later: you are winning at life. Here are your post-workout cool down stretches (see page 144)
>>>>>>

WEEK 2

—

Now we're in week 2, I've got you new workout combinations to keep things interesting and tone your body from all angles.

HERE'S YOUR SCHEDULE:

Monday:	**FULL BODY**
Tuesday:	**BARRE**
Wednesday:	**REST DAY**
Thursday:	**BOXING**
Friday:	**LOWER BODY**
Saturday:	**REST DAY**
Sunday:	**UPPER BODY**

Just as in week 1, you're going to do 45 minutes x 5 days, and each workout involves 6 rounds of HIIT. You can use the same timer you set up for last week as we'll repeat 45 seconds exercise + 15 seconds rest with a 60 second rest between rounds.

If you set your own workout schedule in week 1, try to repeat that rhythm this week so your rest days are spread out.

WARM UP

Here's a quick reminder of the warm up moves:

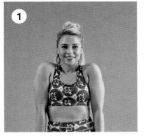

SHOULDER ROLLS

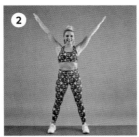

ARM CIRCLES

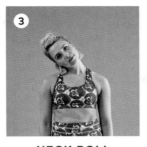

NECK ROLL

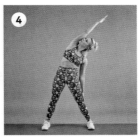

SIDE STRETCH

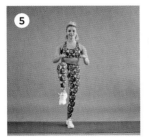

HIGH KNEES

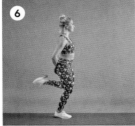

KICK BUTT

COOL DOWN

And another for how to cool down...

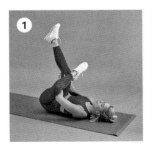

BUTT STRETCH

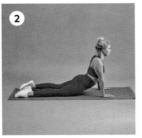

AB STRETCH

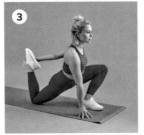

THIGH STRETCH

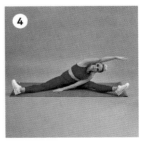

HAMSTRING STRETCH

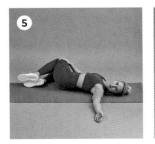

BACK STRETCH

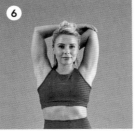

TRICEP STRETCH

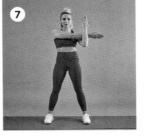

SHOULDER STRETCH

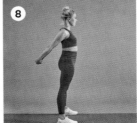

CHEST STRETCH

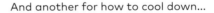

FULL BODY

- Warm up (see page 143)
- 5 combinations, with 15 seconds rest between each combination and 60 seconds rest after each round
- Complete 6 rounds
- Cool down (see page 144)

1. SIDE LUNGES + SQUATS

- From standing, take a wide step into a side lunge, weight in your heel, chest lifted x 1
- Push back to standing then squat x 1
- Lunge to the opposite side x 1
- Push back to standing then squat x 1
- Repeat sequence

2. MOUNTAIN CLIMBERS + SHOULDER TAPS

- Start in high plank position, belly button pulled to spine; straight line from head to heels; shoulders over wrists; pushing floor away to separate shoulders
- Bring alternate knees into chest x 4, keeping hips in line with shoulders
- Tap hand to opposite shoulder x 4
- Repeat sequence

3. JUMPING LUNGES + POP JUMP TOUCH

- Step one leg back into lunge position, belly button pulled to spine, shin parallel to the floor
- Jump, changing legs to land with the opposite leg back
- Do x 4 jumping lunges followed by x 1 pop jump touch
- Repeat sequence

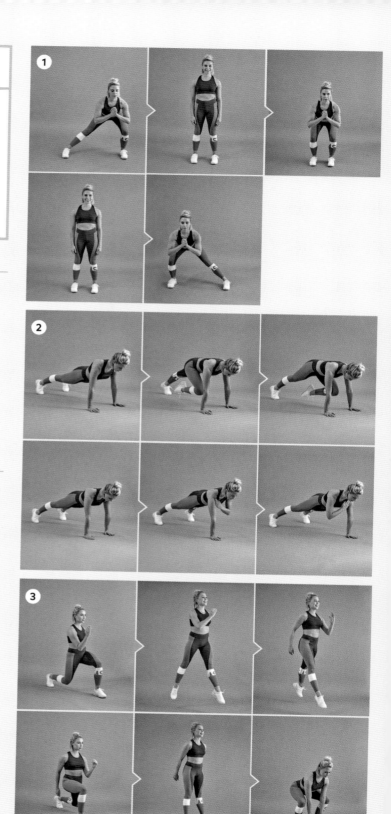

4. JUMPING JACKS + BURPEE

- From standing, do x 4 jumping jacks
- Drop your hands to the floor and jump out to high plank then jump back to standing
- Repeat sequence

5. COMMANDO ELBOWS + PLANK JACKS

- Start in high plank position, belly button pulled to spine
- Come down on to elbows, one arm at a time into elbow plank, keeping your back straight and core tight
- Push up from elbows to palms returning to high plank
- Jump feet out as if you were performing a jumping jack x 4
- Repeat sequence

[Rest for 60 seconds before repeating the full body circuit.]

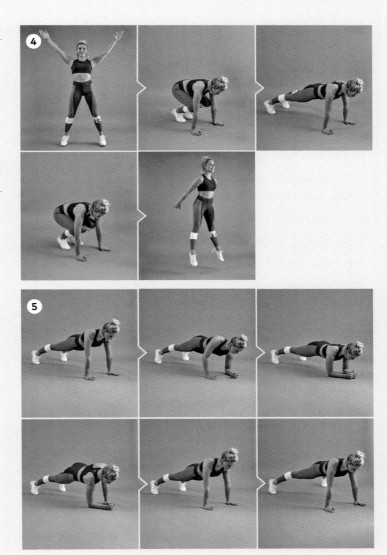

Completed 6 rounds? Boom! Now cool down with your post-workout stretches (see page 144)

>>>>>>

BARRE

- Warm up (see page 143)
- 5 combinations, with 15 seconds rest between each combination and 60 seconds rest after each round
- Complete 6 rounds
- Cool down (see page 144)

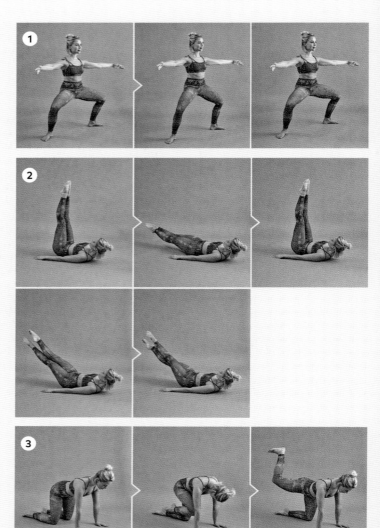

1. PLIÉ HOLD + PULSE

- Start in second position; feet turned out (at 10 to 2); belly button pulled to spine, arms out, shoulders down
- Drop butt down to plié keeping your spine straight; tail bone pointing to the floor (don't arch your back)
- Hold for 4 counts
- Pulse up and down x 4
- Push up to standing
- Repeat sequence

2. LEG LOWER + CRISS CROSS

- Point your toes to the sky (bend your knees if you need to), belly button pulled into spine, head and shoulders lifted
- Lower your legs slowly, as far as you can without arching your back off the floor, then raise back to start position x 4
- Criss cross your legs as you lower slowly and raise to start position x 4
- Repeat sequence

3. DONKEY KICK + CRUNCH

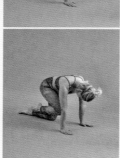

- On all fours, back flat, belly button pulled into spine, shoulders away from ears, slowly crunch one knee to chest then kick the heel back towards the sky without arching your back; squeeze your glutes on the kick
- Keep going! Swap legs at halfway time

4. FIRST + SECOND POSITION JUMPS

- Start in first position; feet turned out (at 10 to 2); belly button pulled to spine, hands on hips, shoulders down
- Plié, knees over toes, tucking your butt so your tail bone points to the floor
- Pushing through the heels, jump and land in second position, bending knees
- Jump again, this time landing back in first position, knees bent
- Repeat sequence. Get jumping, b*tches!

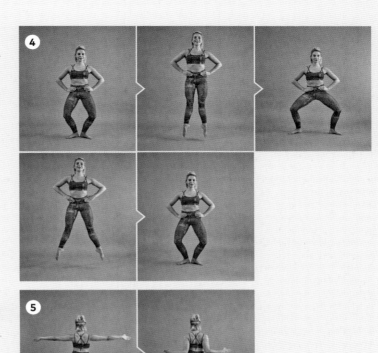

5. PLIÉ HOLD + SHOULDER BLADE SQUEEZE

- Start in second position
- Drop butt down to a deep plié keeping your spine straight; tail bone pointing to the floor (don't arch your back). Hold
- Reach your arms out to second position, keeping your shoulders down and away from your ears
- Slowly squeeze your shoulder blades together, pulling your elbows in then return to second; stay in a deep plié
- Keep going, feel that burn!

[Rest for 60 seconds before repeating the barre circuit.]

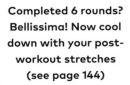

Completed 6 rounds? Bellissima! Now cool down with your post-workout stretches (see page 144)

>>>>>>

BOXING

- Warm up (see page 143)
- 5 combinations, with 15 seconds rest between each combination and 60 seconds rest after each round
- Complete 6 rounds
- Cool down (see page 144)

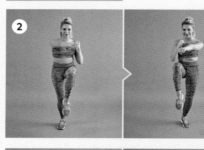

1. REVERSE LUNGE + KICK

– Hands in guard, step one leg back into lunge position, shin parallel to the floor
– Return to standing and kick the opposite leg forward, driving through your heel
– Switch legs at halfway time

2. HIGH KNEES + CROSS

– Run on the spot, lifting knees to hip height
– Pull your belly button into spine as you twist your torso and punch across your body. Keep it up!

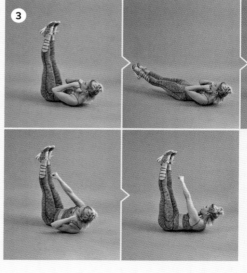

3. LEG LOWER + JABS

– Point your toes to the sky (bend your knees if you need to), head and shoulders lifted, hands in guard position
– Lower your legs slowly, as far as you can without arching your back off the floor, then raise back to start position x 1
– Jab towards your feet with alternate arms x 4
– Repeat sequence

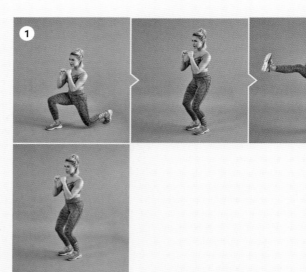

4. SIDE LUNGE + CROSS + POP JUMP

- From standing, in guard position, take a wide step into a side lunge; punch towards the lunging foot with the opposite arm x 1
- Push back to standing; take a pop jump x 1
- Lunge to the opposite side and punch x 1
- Repeat sequence

5. WALKOUT + UPPER CUTS

- Roll down through the spine, walking hands out to high plank position; belly button pulled to spine; straight line from head to heels; shoulders over wrists, pushing floor away to separate shoulders
- Punch uppercuts from underneath x 4, keeping your body as still as possible and your core strong
- Walk hands back in, rolling through the spine to standing
- Repeat sequence

[Rest for 60 seconds before repeating the boxing circuit.]

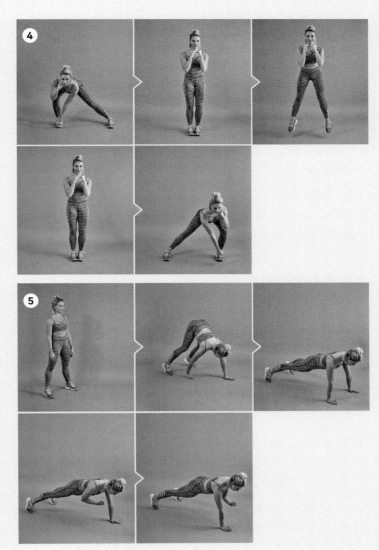

Completed 6 rounds? Game on. Now cool down with your post-workout stretches
(see page 144)
>>>>>>

LOWER BODY

- Warm up (see page 143)
- 5 combinations, with 15 seconds rest between each combination and 60 seconds rest after each round
- Complete 6 rounds
- Cool down (see page 144)

1. FIRE HYDRANT + EXTENSION

- On all fours, back flat, belly button pulled into spine, shoulders away from ears, lift one knee to the side, keeping the knee in line with the hips
- Extend the leg straight out to the side x 1
- Bend the leg back, then lower to starting position, without resting your knee on the floor
- Repeat, switching legs at halfway time

2. LUNGE JUMP + SQUATS

- Step one leg back into lunge position, shin parallel to the floor
- Jump, changing legs to land with the opposite leg back x 4
- Jump again, into a deep squat
- Repeat sequence

3. SPLIT SQUAT

- Rest one foot on the chair behind you (slightly wider than hip width to help you balance)
- Keep your weight in your heel as you lower down into a split squat, then push back to start position, squeezing your glutes at the top
- Switch legs at halfway time

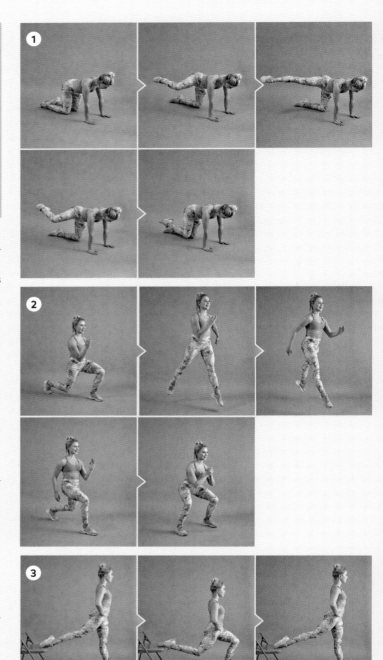

4. BUTT KICK + JUMPING JACK

– This is about speed, go as fast as you can: run on the spot, kicking heels up to butt x 4
– Perform x 4 jumping jacks
– Repeat sequence

5. BUTT BRIDGE + SWING

– Lying on floor, feet hip width apart, heels down, squeezing your butt, pulling belly button into spine, lift your hips to the sky
– Hold for 4 counts
– Squeezing one glute at a time, swing your hips, drawing a half moon shape x 4
– Lower and repeat sequence

[Rest for 60 seconds before repeating the lower body circuit.]

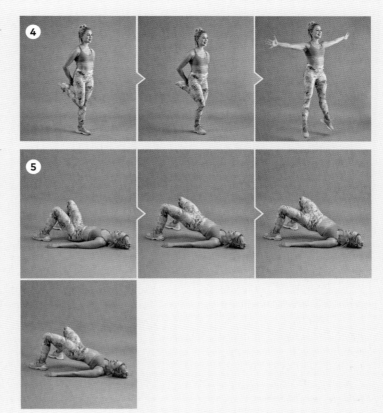

Completed 6 rounds? You rock. Now cool down with your post-workout stretches (see page 144)
>>>>>>

UPPER BODY

- Warm up (see page 143)
- 5 combinations, with 15 seconds rest between each combination and 60 seconds rest after each round
- Complete 6 rounds
- Cool down (see page 144)

1. SIDE PLANK + WRAP

- In side plank, elbow underneath shoulder, belly button pulled into spine, hips lifted off floor, stretch your free arm up and hold x 4 counts (rest on your knee, if needed: see page 170)
- Slowly wrap the straight arm around your body, twisting your torso x 4
- Straighten arm back out and repeat sequence
- Switch sides at halfway time

2. CRISS CROSS ARMS + HALF SQUAT

- Take a wide stance and half squat, reach your arms out in front of you; criss cross arms x 4
- Reach your arms above your head and criss cross them x 4
- Repeat sequence, go faster!

3. COMMANDO PLANK + MOUNTAIN CLIMBERS

- Start in high plank
- Come down on to elbows, one arm at a time into elbow plank; push up from elbows to palms returning to high plank
- Bring alternate knees into chest x 4, keeping hips in line with shoulders
- Repeat sequence

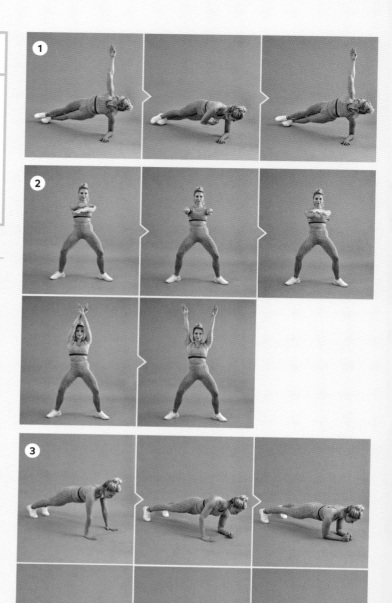

4. TRICEP DIP + TOE REACH

- Weight equally in hands and heels, shoulders away from ears, fingers pointed forward or sideways, elbows tucked in; bend your arms to lower your butt x 4 (make sure your elbows stay pointed out behind you as you bend your arms)
- Straighten arms, then slowly reach an opposite hand to foot, keeping your hips lifted, x 4
- Repeat sequence, swaping hands and feet each time

5. HALF SUPERWOMAN

- Start in high plank
- Lift one leg to hip height, hold x 4 counts, then lower
- Raise the opposite arm and hold x 4 counts
- Repeat with other leg and arm
- Keep going – this one is all about control!

[Rest for 60 seconds before repeating the upper body circuit.]

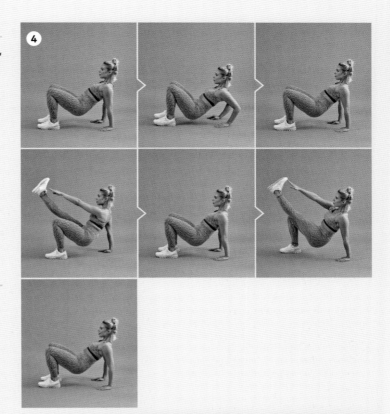

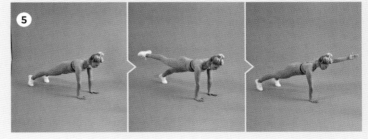

Done 6 rounds? You're amazing! Now lie back, cool down and stretch out...
(see page 144)
>>>>>>

WEEK 3

Now you've built up a strong base of fitness, you're going to step up to 5 sessions x 60 minutes. That 60 minutes includes your warm up and cool down, so it's totally doable.

HERE'S YOUR SCHEDULE:

Monday:	**FULL BODY**
Tuesday:	**BARRE**
Wednesday:	**REST DAY**
Thursday:	**BOXING**
Friday:	**LOWER BODY**
Saturday:	**REST DAY**
Sunday:	**UPPER BODY**

Adjust your timer.

In each workout this week, you'll do 6 different exercise combinations of 45 seconds each, with 15 seconds rest between each combination. That's one round.

You've got a 60 second rest interval before you repeat the round.

You'll complete 6 rounds in total.

WARM UP

Here's a quick reminder of the warm up moves:

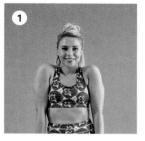
SHOULDER ROLLS

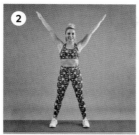
ARM CIRCLES

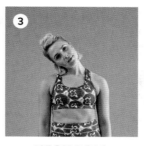
NECK ROLL

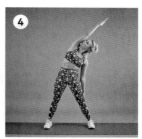
SIDE STRETCH

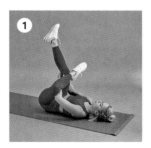
HIGH KNEES

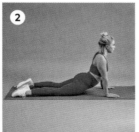
KICK BUTT

COOL DOWN

And another for how to cool down...

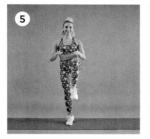
BUTT STRETCH

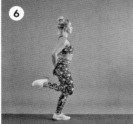
AB STRETCH

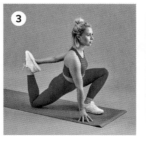
THIGH STRETCH

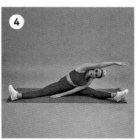
HAMSTRING STRETCH

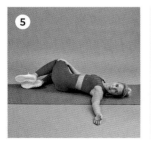
BACK STRETCH

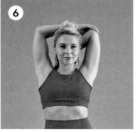
TRICEP STRETCH

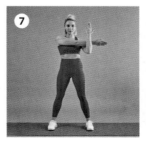
SHOULDER STRETCH

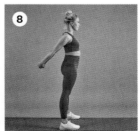
CHEST STRETCH

FULL BODY

- Warm up (see page 143)
- 6 combinations, with 15 seconds rest between each combination and 60 seconds rest after each round
- Complete 6 rounds
- Cool down (see page 144)

1. WALKOUT + HALF BURPEE

- Roll down through the spine, walking hands out to high plank
- Jump feet in towards your chest for a half burpee, then straight back out
- Walk hands back to standing position
- Repeat sequence with speed!

2. MOUNTAIN CLIMBERS CROSS + SHOULDER TAPS

- Start in high plank; straight line from head to heels; shoulders over wrists; pushing floor away to separate shoulders
- Slowly cross each knee to the opposite elbow x 4
- Tap each hand to the opposite shoulder x 4
- Repeat sequence

3. SIDE PLANK WRAPS + PULSE

- In side plank, elbow underneath shoulder, belly button pulled into spine, hips lifted off floor, stretch your free arm up and hold x 4 counts (see knee variation)
- Slowly wrap the straight arm around your body, twisting your torso x 4
- Pulse your hips to the sky x 4 then switch sides at halfway time

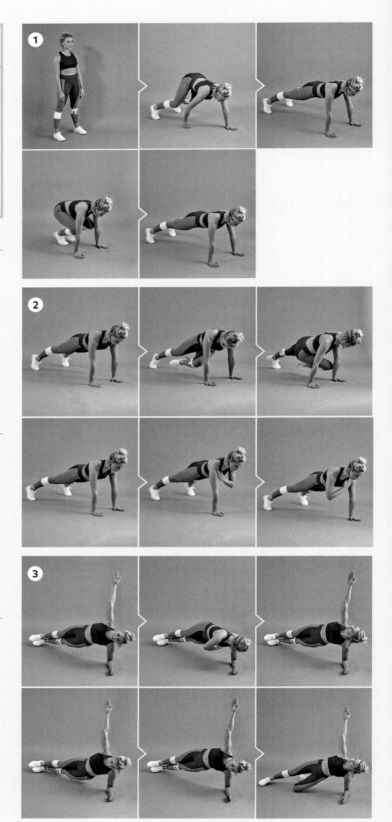

4. KNEE DRIVES + HOP

- Step one leg back into lunge position, shin parallel to the floor
- Push through the back leg as you drive the knee forward into a hop
- Take the same leg back to lunge, switching legs at halfway time. This is about power!

5. CRAB PLANK + CRAB WALK

- On all fours, back flat, belly button pulled into spine, shoulders away from ears, raise knees off the ground, then walk hands and feet four steps left
- Hold x 4 counts, then step hands and feet four steps right, back to start position; hold x 4 counts
- Repeat sequence

6. LONG JUMP + MONSTER WALK

- Feet hip width apart, take a big jump forwards landing in a deep squat
- Stay in squat position and take big steps back to your starting position
- Stand up and repeat sequence

[Rest for 60 seconds before repeating the full body circuit.]

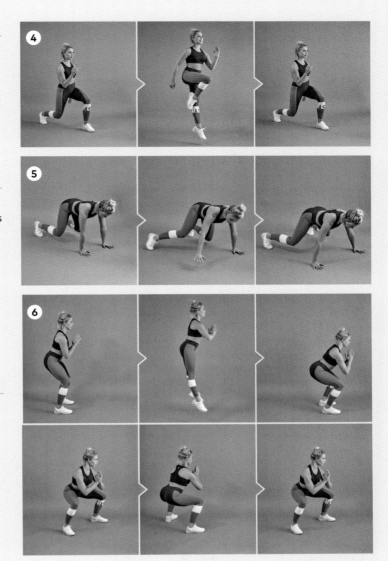

Completed 6 rounds? Wow! Now cool down with your post-workout stretches (see page 144)
>>>>>>

BARRE

- Warm up (see page 143)
- 6 combinations, with 15 seconds rest between each combination and 60 seconds rest after each round
- Complete 6 rounds
- Cool down (see page 144)

1. PLIÉ + HEEL RAISE

- Start in second position; feet turned out (at 10 to 2); belly button pulled to spine, arms out, shoulders down
- Drop butt down to a deep plié keeping your spine straight; tail bone pointing to the floor (don't arch your back). Hold
- Raise your heels as if you're wearing your highest stilettos. Higher!
- Lower heels to floor and straighten legs
- Repeat sequence

2. BEND + SQUEEZE

- Reach one arm up to the sky as you reach the other hand down towards the knee
- Squeeze your ribs to hips as you bend to one side. Count 4 on the way down and 4 on the way back to standing
- Repeat, switching sides at halfway time

3. ARABESQUE + PULSE

- From standing, legs slightly bent (don't lock knees), use your glute and hamstring to raise one leg up and hold x 4
- Then pulse up x 4. Try not to rest toe on the floor between lifts
- Switch to the other leg at halfway time

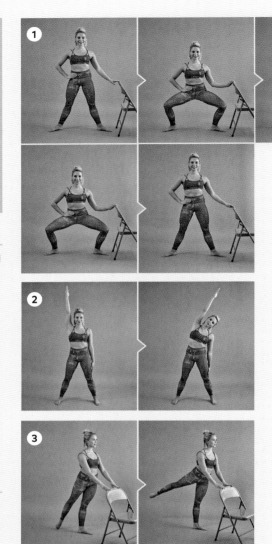

4. LEG LOWER + ARMS TO FIFTH

- Point toes to the sky (bend your knees if you need to), belly button pulled into spine, head and shoulders lifted, arms reaching up
- Lower your legs and arms as low as you can go without arching your back off the floor x 1
- Raise back up to start position, crunching and reaching hands to feet x 4
- Repeat sequence

5. CLAM OPEN + TOUCH

- Lying on your side, extend your top arm and leg out, toes pointed
- Squeeze your elbow to knee, ribs to hips, to work the obliques x 1
- Lift and lengthen the arm and leg back out
- Repeat sequence switching sides at halfway time

6. PLIÉ JUMPS + ARMS IN FIFTH

- Start in second position; feet turned out (at 10 to 2), shoulders down, arms raised to fifth position
- Drop butt down to a deep plié keeping your spine straight
- Jump, pushing through your heels, and land with soft knees, heels to floor.
- Repeat sequence, arms raised throughout!

[Rest for 60 seconds before repeating the barre circuit.]

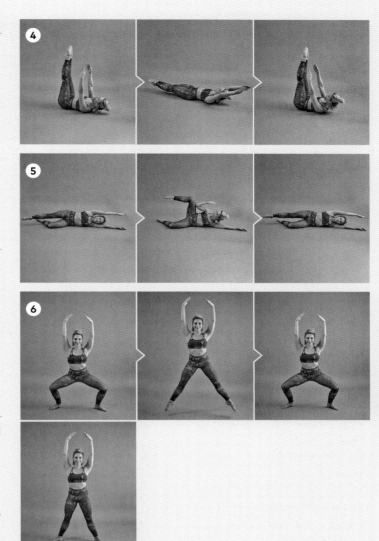

Completed 6 rounds? Champ! Now cool down with your post-workout stretches.
(see page 144)

BOXING

- Warm up (see page 143)
- 6 combinations, with 15 seconds rest between each combination and 60 seconds rest after each round
- Complete 6 rounds
- Cool down (see page 144)

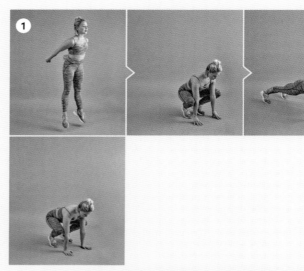

1. LONG JUMP BURPEE + 180°

– Feet hip width apart, take a big jump forwards
– Drop your hands to the floor and jump out to high plank
– Jump feet back in
– Jump to standing, turning 180° to face in the opposite direction and repeat the sequence

2. ELBOW PLANK + HALF MOONS

– Start in elbow plank position, elbows under shoulders, forearms planted, straight line from head to heels. Hold for 4 counts
– Dip one hip at a time, creating a half moon shape x 4.
– Repeat sequence

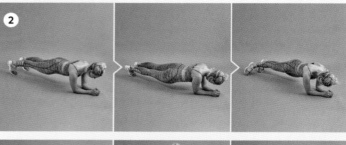

3. SQUAT JUMP + JABS

– From a wide stance, jump into a deep squat keeping your chest up, weight in heels and guard up x 4
– Hold the last squat down and jab with each arm x 4
– Repeat sequence

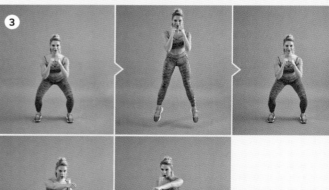

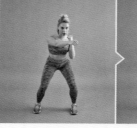

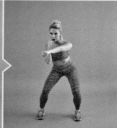

4. FROGGERS + UPPER CUTS

- From a wide stance, jump into a high plank; jump feet to replace hands, lifting chest and keeping the butt low, so you look like a frog. Ribbet
- Drop your hands again and jump feet back out into high plank x 2
- Hold the second squat and perform x 4 uppercuts
- Repeat sequence, feel that burn!

5. SIDE LUNGE + TORSO TWIST

- From standing, take a wide step into a side lunge, weight in your heel, chest lifted
- Push through the bent leg to drive the knee up and twist the torso towards the lifted leg
- Repeat sequence, swapping legs at halfway time

6. ROCKING JABS + POP JUMP TOUCH

- From a wide stance, rock from foot to foot, jabbing forward x 4
- Pop jump up and land touching the floor x 1
- Repeat sequence

[Rest for 60 seconds before repeating the boxing circuit.]

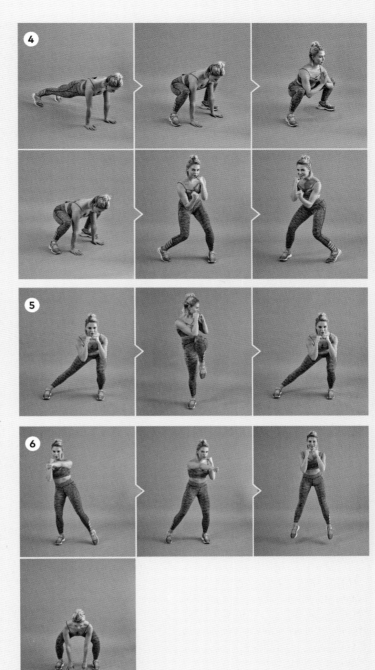

Completed 6 rounds? Brilliant! Now it's time to stretch and cool down (see page 144)

>>>>>>

LOWER BODY

- Warm up (see page 143)
- 6 combinations, with 15 seconds rest between each combination and 60 seconds rest after each round
- Complete 6 rounds
- Cool down (see page 144)

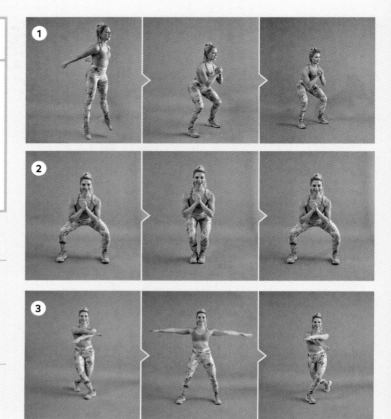

1. LONG JUMP FORWARD + BOUNCE BACKS

- Feet hip width apart, take a big jump forwards
- Bounce back to start position
- Repeat sequence

2. SQUAT HOLD + WALKS

- From standing, feet wide, squat and hold for 4 counts
- Step sideways x 2. Hold x 4
- Step sideways in the opposite direction x 2. Hold x 4
- Repeat sequence

3. CURTSEY LUNGE + CRISS CROSS ARMS

- From standing, curtsey one leg back and behind, bending the knees into a deep lunge, keeping knees in line with toes
- Hold the curtsey lunge and criss cross arms x 4
- Push up, step to the opposite side and curtsey lunge with the other leg, criss crossing arms x 4
- Repeat sequence

4. BUTT BRIDGE + LEG EXTENSION

- Lying on floor, feet hip width apart, heels down, squeezing your butt, lift your hips to the sky and hold x 4 counts
- Extend one leg, keeping your hips lifted and square. Hold x 4
- Lower the leg and hold the bridge x 4
- Extend the other leg and hold x 4
- Repeat sequence

5. IN/OUT SQUATS + TOUCHDOWN

- Starting in a wide squat position, jump into a narrow squat, then back out into a wide squat
- Touch the floor with your hands
- Repeat sequence

6. FIRE HYDRANT EXTENSION + TOE TAPS

- On all fours, back flat, belly button pulled into spine, shoulders away from ears, extend one leg to the side, toe resting on the floor
- Squeeze your glutes, slowly lift the extended leg up and down
- Repeat sequence
- Switch legs at halfway time

[Rest for 60 seconds before repeating the lower body circuit.]

Smashed 6 rounds? Amazing! Now cool down with your post-workout stretches (see page 144)

>>>>>>

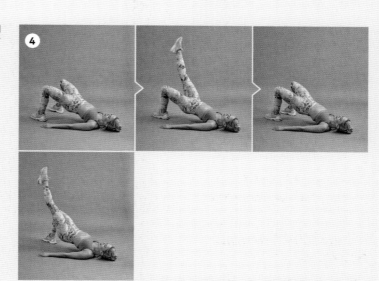

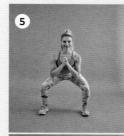
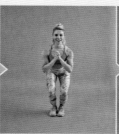
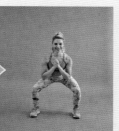
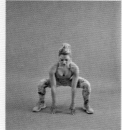
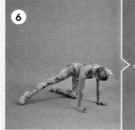
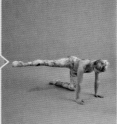

UPPER BODY

- Warm up (see page 143)
- 6 combinations, with 15 seconds rest between each combination and 60 seconds rest after each round
- Complete 6 rounds
- Cool down (see page 144)

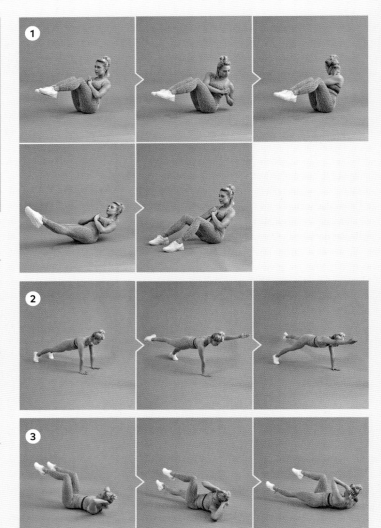

1. RUSSIAN TWISTS + LEG EXTENSION

– With legs in table top (or feet on floor), belly button pulled into spine, hands clasped in front of your chest, twist your shoulders and hands to each side x 4
– Return to centre, then extend your legs and lower your back halfway to the floor x 1. Return to start position and repeat sequence

2. SUPERWOMAN ARMS + LEGS

– Start in high plank; straight line from head to heels; shoulders over wrists; pushing floor away to separate shoulders
– Slowly raise one arm and the opposite leg. Find your balance
– Return to high plank then raise the other arm and leg
– Repeat sequence

3. BICYCLE CRUNCHES FAST + SLOW

– Start with legs in table top, hands behind ears, head and shoulders lifted
– With control, slowly move one elbow to opposite knee, as the other leg extends x 4
– Then pick up the pace x 4
– Repeat sequence

4. WALKOUT + PRESS

- Roll down through the spine, walking hands out to high plank position; belly button pulled to spine; straight line from head to heels; shoulders over wrists, pushing floor away to separate shoulders
- Press to lower your chest to the floor, keeping back straight (press on knees if you need to)
- Push up and walk hands back to feet, roll up to stand
- Repeat sequence

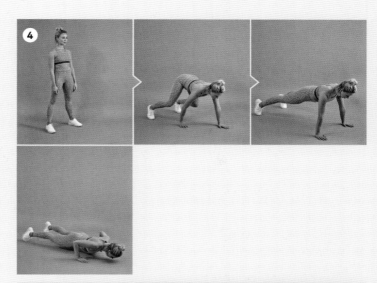

5. BACK LIFT + SWIM

- Start on your front, with arms and legs extended
- Pull belly button into spine, lift arms and legs off the floor. Hold
- Lift an arm and opposite leg higher. Then repeat with the other arm and leg x 4
- Lower to the floor then repeat sequence

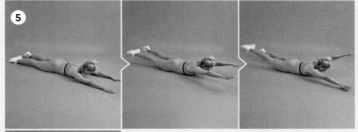
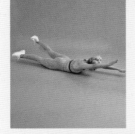

6. BEAR CRAWL FORWARD + BACK

- On all fours, in crawl position, keeping your back parallel to the floor, crawl hands and feet forwards x 4
- Crawl back x 4
- Repeat sequence

[Rest for 60 seconds before repeating the upper body circuit.]

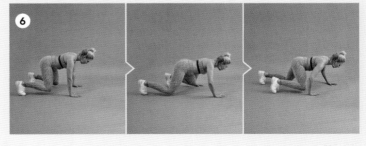

Sweat flying off you after 6 rounds? You're getting results already! Now cool down with your post-workout stretches (see page 144)

>>>>>>

WEEK 4

You made it to week 4! Now we're going to seriously shape up with another 5 sessions x 60 minutes. From warm up to cool down, your whole workout is done and dusted in an hour.

HERE'S YOUR SCHEDULE:

Monday:	**FULL BODY**
Tuesday:	**BARRE**
Wednesday:	**REST DAY**
Thursday:	**BOXING**
Friday:	**LOWER BODY**
Saturday:	**REST DAY**
Sunday:	**UPPER BODY**

WARM UP

Here's a quick reminder of the warm up moves:

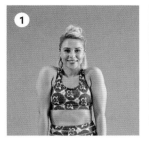

1 SHOULDER ROLLS

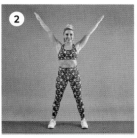

2 ARM CIRCLES

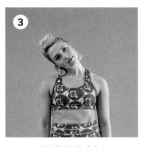

3 NECK ROLL

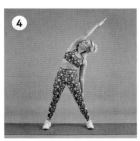

4 SIDE STRETCH

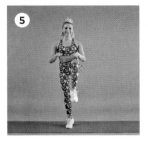

5 HIGH KNEES

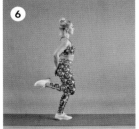

6 KICK BUTT

COOL DOWN

And another for how to cool down...

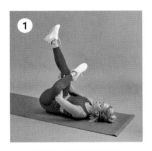

1 BUTT STRETCH

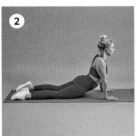

2 AB STRETCH

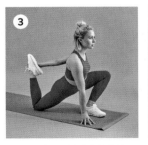

3 THIGH STRETCH

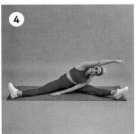

4 HAMSTRING STRETCH

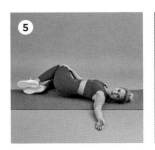

5 BACK STRETCH

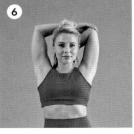

6 TRICEP STRETCH

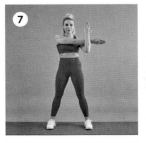

7 SHOULDER STRETCH

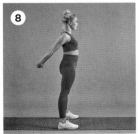

8 CHEST STRETCH

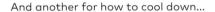

FULL BODY

- Warm up (see page 143)
- 6 combinations, with 15 seconds rest between each combination and 60 seconds rest after each round
- Complete 6 rounds
- Cool down (see page 144)

1. CRAB PLANK + KICK THROUGH

- On all fours, back flat, belly button pulled into spine, shoulders away from ears, raise knees an inch
- Kick one foot through to the opposite side, dropping your hips and releasing the opposite hand
- Repeat on the other side
- Continue to the beep, b*tches!

2. OUT/IN JUMPS + BURPEE

- Starting in a wide squat position, jump into a narrow squat, then back out into a wide squat
- Drop hands to floor and jump out to high plank
- Jump feet forward to hands and jump up to stand
- Repeat sequence!

3. SUPERWOMAN + ELBOW TO KNEE

- Start in high plank, belly button pulled to spine; straight line from head to heels; shoulders over wrists; pushing floor away to separate shoulders
- Slowly extend one arm and the opposite leg. Find your balance
- With control, bring elbow and knee to touch
- Return to start position and swap sides
- Repeat sequence

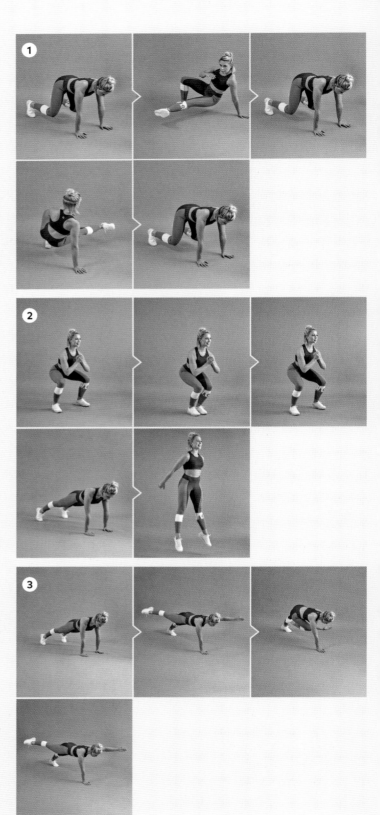

4. CRAB PLANK + BUNNY HOP

- On all fours, back flat, belly button pulled into spine, shoulders away from ears, raise knees off the ground. Hold x 4 counts
- Push through your feet to lift your hips up, keeping knees bent x 2
- Return to crab plank position and repeat sequence. Do not let your knees touch the floor!!

5. ELBOW PLANK + SAW

- Start in elbow plank, elbows under shoulders, forearms planted, straight line from head to heels
- Slow and controlled, rock your weight forward towards your hands, then back to start position
- Repeat sequence

6. SKATERS + SQUAT JUMPS

- From standing, jump to the side landing on one foot, swinging the other leg behind you as if you were rollerblading down Venice Beach
- Jump to the other side, repeating the move x 4
- Follow this move up with x 4 squat jumps!
- Repeat sequence

[Rest for 60 seconds before repeating the full body circuit.]

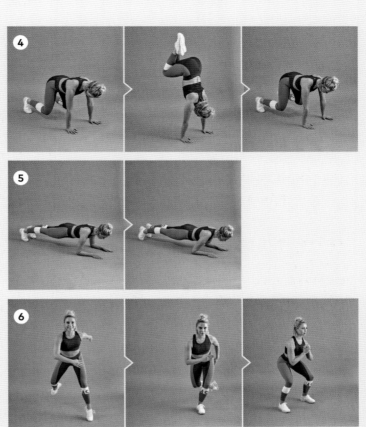

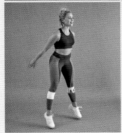

FULL BODY

WEEK 4

Completed 6 rounds? You're amazing! Now cool down with your post-workout stretches (see page 144)
>>>>>>

BARRE

- Warm up (see page 143)
- 5 combinations, with 15 seconds rest between each combination and 60 seconds rest after each round
- Complete 6 rounds
- Cool down (see page 144)

1. PLIÉ + KNEE TO ELBOW

- Start in second position; feet turned out (at 10 to 2); belly button pulled to spine, one arm reaching into fifth position, shoulders down
- Drop butt to a deep plié keeping spine straight (don't arch). Hold
- As you rise up, bring one elbow to knee, squeezing ribs to hips, to engage your obliques
- Repeat sequence, returning to full plié between each oblique lift
- Swap sides at halfway time

2. BARRE SKATERS + PLIÉ JUMPS

- From standing, jump to one side, landing on one foot, swinging the other leg behind you; keep arms up and supported, one in front and one to the side; then jump to the other side x 4
- Now jump in first position x 4
- Repeat sequence, at speed!!!

3. AB CRUNCH + LEG EXTENSION

- Lying on your side, extend your top arm and leg out, toes pointed
- Crunch your abdominals to lift your extended leg out in front of you and reach your extended arm towards your toe.
- Return to start position and repeat sequence
- Switch sides at halfway time

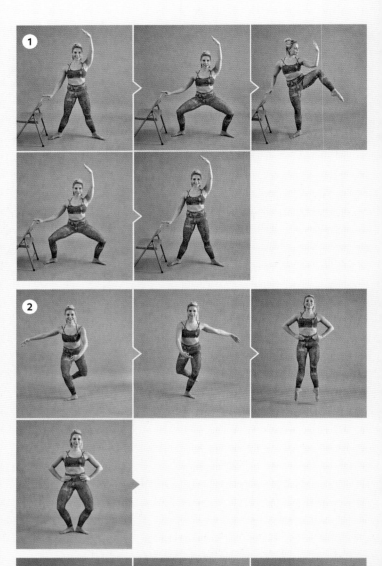

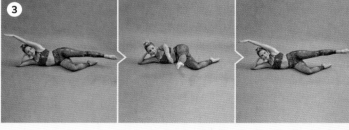

4. PLIÉ LIFT + SHOULDER BLADE SQUEEZE

- Start in second position; feet turned out; belly button to spine, shoulders down
- Drop butt down to a deep plié keeping spine straight. Hold
- Staying in your plié, raise and lower your heels x 4
- Hold the last raise up and stretch your free arm out. Squeeze your shoulder blades together, bringing your elbows in x 4
- Repeat sequence, switching sides at halfway time

5. AB CRUNCH + SCISSOR LEGS

- Point toes to the sky (bend knees if you need to), head and shoulders lifted, hands behind ears.
- Turn knees out to engage inner thighs
- Crunch up x 4
- Lower your legs as far as you can go without arching your back, scissoring legs with control x 4
- Repeat sequence

6. TINY ARM CIRCLES + PLIÉ

- Start in second position; feet turned out; belly button to spine, shoulders down
- Drop butt down to a deep plié keeping spine straight; tail bone pointing to the floor (don't arch). Hold
- Reach your arms out to the side. Circle your arms forward x 4 then back x 4
- Stay in deep plié throughout, feel that burn...

[Rest for 60 seconds before repeating the barre circuit.]

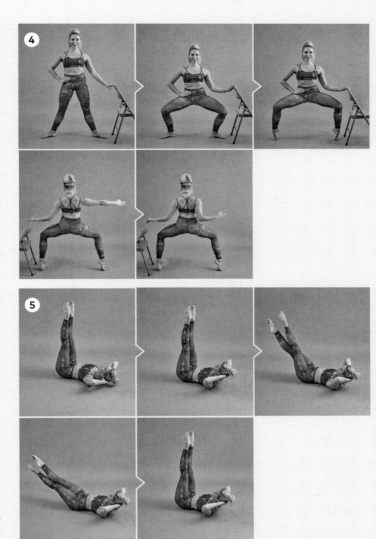

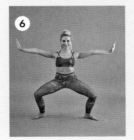

Completed 6 rounds? Total hero! Now cool down with your post-workout stretches (see page 144)

>>>>>>

BOXING

- Warm up (see page 143)
- 6 combinations, with 15 seconds rest between each combination and 60 seconds rest after each round
- Complete 6 rounds
- Cool down (see page 144)

1. SQUAT JUMP + HOOK

- From a wide stance, perform x 4 squat jumps, keeping your guard up
- Punch as though you are trying to hit someone in the ribs, using your torso to get power into each punch x 4
- Repeat sequence

2. SHOULDER TAP + FROGGER

- Start in high plank
- Tap each hand to the opposite shoulder x 4. Repeat sequence
- Jump feet to replace hands, lifting chest and keeping the butt low, so you look like a frog x 4
- Repeat sequence

3. HALF MOON HIPS + OBLIQUE KNEE LIFT

- Start in elbow plank, elbows under shoulders, forearms planted, straight line from head to heels
- Dip one hip at a time, creating a half moon shape x 4
- Bring knee to elbow x 4
- Repeat sequence, swapping legs each time

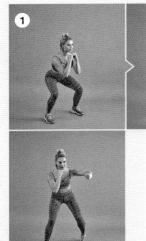
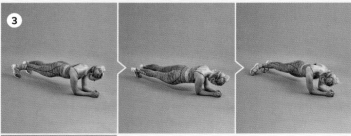
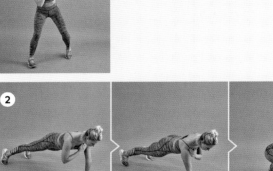
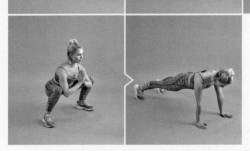
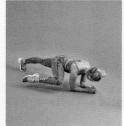

4. POP JUMP TOUCH + ROCKING JABS

- From standing, jump up, bending the legs as you land and drop hands to touch floor x 4
- Rock from foot to foot, jabbing forward x 4
- Repeat sequence

5. LUNGE JUMP + KICKS

- Hands in guard position, step one leg back into lunge position, belly button pulled to spine, shin parallel to floor
- Jump, landing back on the opposite back leg x 4
- Bring your back leg back in, then kick forward with the opposite leg, driving through the heel. Repeat, kicking with the same leg, x 4
- Repeat sequence, changing legs for the kick each time

6. ROCKING HOOKS + UPPERCUTS

- From a wide stance, rock from side to side, staying on your toes
- Hook your punches, as if you're trying to punch someone in the ribs x 4
- Keep rocking as you take x 4 uppercut punches, as if you're going for under their ribs
- Repeat sequence

[Rest for 60 seconds before repeating the boxing circuit.]

Completed 6 rounds? You're a knockout! Now cool down with your post-workout stretches (see page 144)
>>>>>>

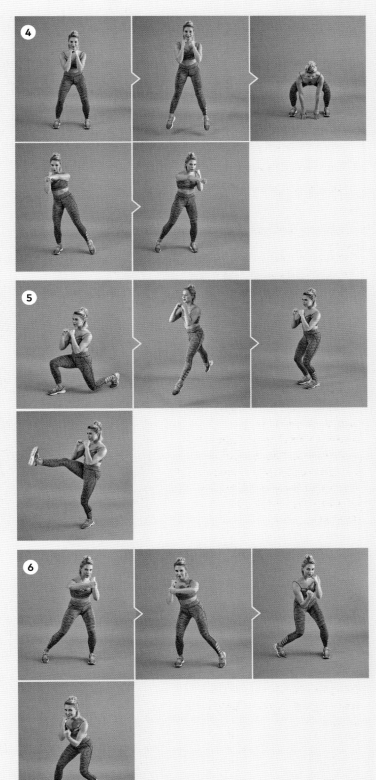

LOWER BODY

- Warm up (see page 143)
- 6 combinations, with 15 seconds rest between each combination and 60 seconds rest after each round
- Complete 6 rounds
- Cool down (see page 144)

1. CURTSEY LUNGES + JUMP SQUAT

- From standing, curtsey one leg behind the other, into a deep lunge. Switch legs, and repeat x 4
- Return to centre and squat jump x 4, as quick as you can
- Repeat sequence

2. KNEE DRIVE + LUNGE PULSE

- Step back into a lunge, belly button pulled to spine, shin parallel to the floor
- Push through the back leg as you drive knee forward to hop x 4
- On the last lunge, hold the lunge down and pulse x 4
- Repeat sequence, switching sides at halfway time

3. FIRE HYDRANT EXTENSION + CROSS TOE TAPS

- On all fours, back flat, shoulders away from ears, extend one leg to the side, toe resting on the floor
- Squeeze your glutes, lift the extended leg up and over the opposite leg, working the inner thigh
- Switch legs at halfway time

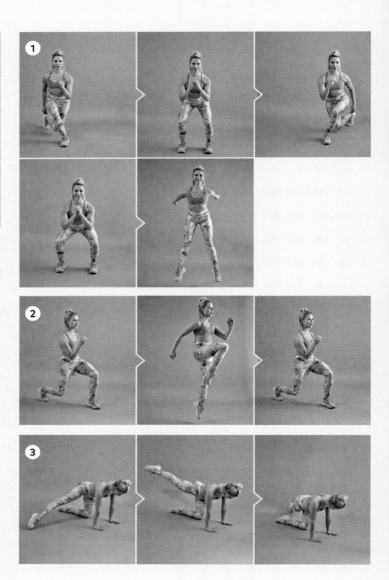

4. LONG JUMP BURPEE + MONSTER WALK

- Jump forward, as far as you can. Land in a deep squat, chest up, weight in heels
- Drop hands, jump feet back to high plank, jump feet back in
- Squat jump x 1
- Stay low in your squat and walk back to start position

5. ELBOW PLANK + LEG LIFT PULSE

- Start in elbow plank, elbows under shoulders, forearms planted, straight line from head to heels
- Raise one foot and pulse the heel up. Keep going till halfway time then swap legs!

6. SQUAT + HALFWAY HOLD

- From a wide stance, squat, keeping chest up and weight in your heels
- Rise up halfway and hold x 4 counts
- Drop back down into deep squat x 4 counts
- Squeeze your butt to return to standing
- Repeat sequence

[Rest for 60 seconds before repeating the lower body circuit.]

Smashed 6 rounds? Awesome! Now bring on the cool down stretches (see page 144)
>>>>>>

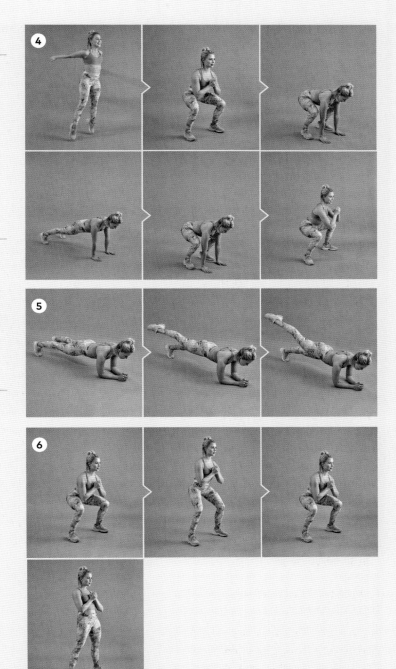

UPPER BODY

- Warm up (see page 143)
- 6 combinations, with 15 seconds rest between each combination and 60 seconds rest after each round
- Complete 6 rounds
- Cool down (see page 144)

1. PLANK + ROTATION

- Start in elbow plank, elbows under shoulders, forearms planted, straight line from head to heels
- Keeping hips lifted, reach one arm to the sky, turning your body to side plank
- Return to elbow plank then repeat the rotation on the other side
- Keep going with control

2. TRICEP DIP + PULSE

- Weight equally in hands and heels, fingers pointing forward or sideways, shoulders away from ears, elbows tucked in, bend arms to lower your butt x 4
- Make sure your elbows stay pointed behind you
- Hold the last dip down and pulse up x 4
- Push back to starting position and repeat sequence

3. CRUNCH + LENGTHEN

- Crunch your head and shoulders and pull in your knees, making yourself as compact as you can
- Reach arms and legs out, making yourself as long as you can. Keep control
- Repeat sequence

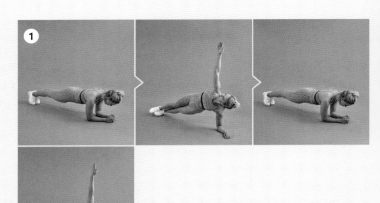

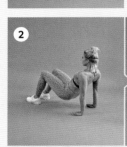

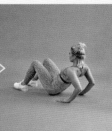
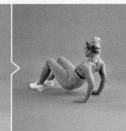

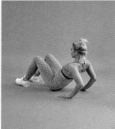

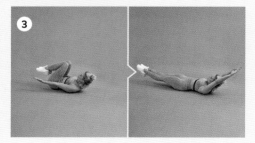

4. PRESS + MOUNTAIN CLIMBER

- Start in high plank
- Bend elbows to lower chest to the floor, keeping back straight x 2
- After the second press, bring alternate knees into chest x 4; keeping hips in line with shoulders. Pick up the speed here, kids!

5. WALKOUTS + HALF SUPERWOMAN

- Roll down through the spine, walking hands out to high plank
- Lift one arm out to half superwoman then return it
- Walk hands back in, rolling up to stand
- Do x 1 pop jump
- Repeat, lifting the other arm

6. ELBOW PLANK + DOLPHIN RAISE

- Start in elbow plank
- Using your core, with control, lift your hips to the sky. Hold for 4 counts
- Lower back to elbow plank
- Repeat sequence

[Rest for 60 seconds before repeating the upper body circuit.]

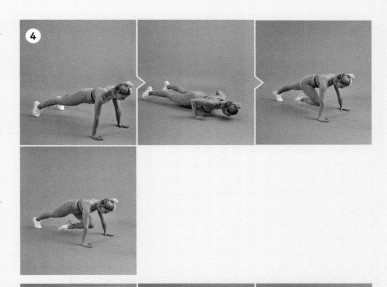

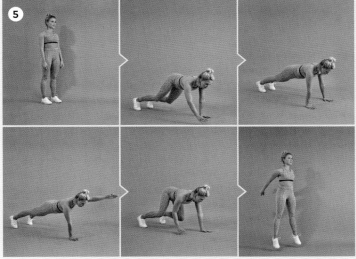

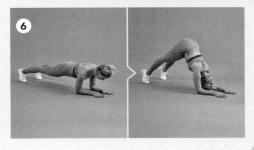

Completed 6 rounds? And nailed 4 weeks of workouts? You are GOLD. Luxuriate in a nice rest and cool down with your post-workout stretches (see page 144)

>>>>>>

Congratulations!

I'm so proud of you. Wow!

Every week you've got fitter, I hope you feel amazing. But what happens now?

What you've got here in this book is a sustainable plan you can keep coming back to. How do I know? Because this is what I do all the time. If you eat well, you can get away with skipping the odd workout. And vice versa: if you eat something a bit crap, really challenge yourself in your next workout. I'll be here to keep cheering you on.

In the last four weeks you've developed the routine and motivation to stay in shape. I hope exercise and eating well is more ingrained in your daily life. Remember how much your body has changed. Here's how to continue your good work:

Send me your recreations of your favourite recipes on Instagram, tagging your photos #shapeupwithgabbyallen

You've got the idea of healthy fast food: protein, veggies, and make it quick. So I'd love you to suggest ideas to me too. Or invite me round for dinner!

Keep up the workouts and keep challenging yourself. Record how many reps you do and monitor your ongoing progress. Share your progress with me on Instagram using #shapeupwithgabbyallen so I can find you.

Shorten your rest time between rounds to 45 seconds instead of 60, or add in an extra round, or an extra combination. My favourite combination has to involve a burpee, every time. I know: psycho! What's your favourite exercise? Let me know.

Alongside the workouts in this book, take a class, weight train or enter a race to keep challenging yourself.

Thank you.

Gabby
xx